Zen at Your Desk

A Guide to Sitting Yoga and Mindful Breathing for Busy Professionals
The Health Secret Hidden in Your Chair.

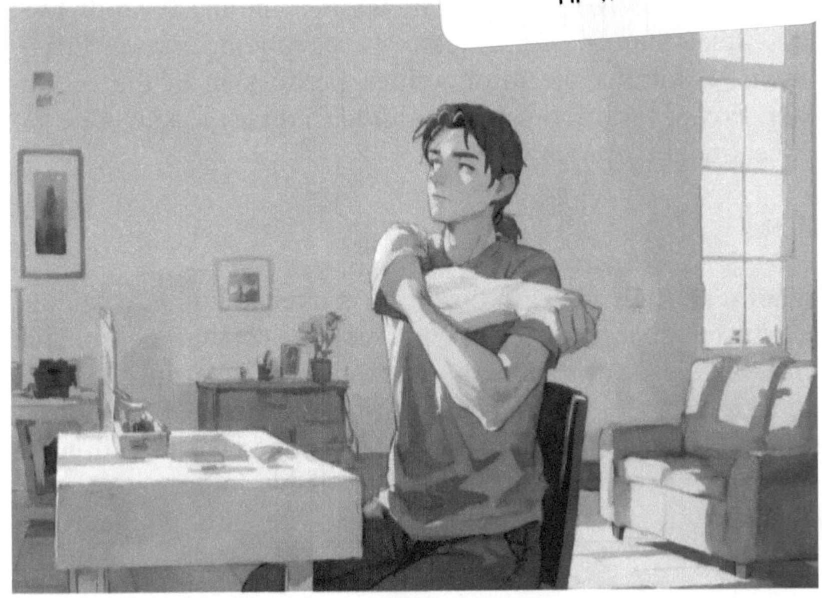

By Jayanta Sarkar

Published by Self-Published
First Edition – 2025

Copyright Page for Zen at Your Desk

Disclaimer: The content in this book is intended for educational and informational purposes only. It is not a substitute for medical advice, diagnosis, or treatment. Readers should consult a qualified healthcare provider before beginning any new fitness, yoga, or breathing routine, especially if they have a medical condition or injury. The author and publisher are not liable for any adverse effects resulting from the use or misuse of the information in this book.

Published By: Self-published by Jayanta Sarkar
Printed In: India

First Edition: March-2025

Contents

Acknowledgments

I am deeply thankful for the guidance of mentors, the support of loved ones specially my daughter Jasmita Sarkar, and the ancient wisdom of yoga, which inspires this work. This book is written with a commitment to the well-being of all beings.

Dedication

Dedicated to all those who spend long hours at their desks yet dream of inner peace. May you find stillness in movement and mindfulness in every breath.

Foreword

In today's fast-paced digital world, the boundaries between work and well-being have become increasingly blurred. As an IT professional, I have witnessed firsthand how long hours at a desk can take a toll on physical health, mental clarity, and overall happiness. Stress, fatigue, and musculoskeletal discomfort have become silent companions for many who spend their days in front of screens. Yet, amid these challenges, a simple yet powerful solution exists—yoga.

Zen at Your Desk is not just another yoga book. It is a practical guide designed specifically for professionals who may not have the luxury of time to step away from their workstations. Through carefully curated sitting yoga poses, this book introduces an accessible approach to wellness—one that fits seamlessly into the workday without requiring extra space, special attire, or elaborate routines.

The brilliance of this book lies in its simplicity. By integrating short, mindful movements and breathing exercises into daily work life, anyone can alleviate stress, improve posture, and enhance focus. These small but powerful changes lead to a profound shift—helping individuals transform their desks from sources of strain into spaces of renewal.

I wholeheartedly believe that well-being should not be a luxury—it should be an integral part of our everyday lives, including our work. Whether you are a software developer, manager, or entrepreneur, Zen at Your Desk offers a path to balance and vitality without disrupting your workflow.

I invite you to explore these practices with an open mind and a willing heart. A few moments of mindful movement can make all the difference. Let this book be your guide to greater ease, resilience, and presence—even in the busiest of workdays.

Jayanta Sarkar
Author, IT Professional & Yoga Practitioner

Preface

In today's fast-paced professional landscape, achieving occupational well-being has become more essential than ever. Balancing the demands of career with personal health requires a mindful approach to physical, mental, and emotional wellness.

Yoga, an ancient practice, offers a transformative path to holistic health. Beyond enhancing physical fitness, it fosters mental clarity, emotional resilience, and improved productivity qualities indispensable in modern workplaces. This book brings these benefits directly to your desk, helping you integrate, simple yet effective yoga practices, which include sitting asana, pranayama and mudra into your daily routine.

Introduction

Finding Balance in a Chaotic World

In today's fast-paced world, relentless technological advancements, global connectivity, and ever-increasing work demands have made occupational well-being a critical imperative for individuals and organizations alike. The modern workplace, filled with constant pressures and stressors, challenges our ability to maintain a healthy work-life balance and holistic well-being.

Many of us spend countless hours hunched over desks, rushing from one deadline to the next, unaware of the gradual toll this lifestyle takes on our bodies and minds. From nagging back pain and stiff shoulders to mental fatigue and dwindling focus, the workplace often feels like a breeding ground for stress and discomfort.

But what if there were a way to reclaim your health and vitality—right from your desk? Imagine weaving moments of calm, clarity, and rejuvenation into your daily routine, all without stepping away from your chair. This book introduces the transformative power of sitting yoga, empowering you to rediscover balance in the midst of your busy work life

The Power of Sitting Yoga

Yoga has long been celebrated for its ability to harmonize the body, mind, and spirit. Yet, in its essence, yoga is not confined to mats or studios. Its principles can be adapted to meet the realities of our lives, no matter where we are. Sitting yoga, a simple and accessible form of yoga, brings the transformative benefits of this ancient practice to the modern workplace.
This book is a guide to practical, effective yoga routines designed to fit seamlessly into your daily work life. Whether you're a seasoned yogi or completely new to the practice, you'll discover exercises and techniques that require no special equipment, no extra space—just your willingness to pause and breathe.

The word "yoga" comes from a Sanskrit root "yuj" which means union, or yoke, to join, and to direct and concentrate one's attention. The yoga Sutra of Patanjali, is considered as the basic text of yoga. These sutras propound the 'ashtanga yoga'. In Patanjali yoga sutra Maharishi Patanjali has described yoga as "योग: चित्त वृत्ति निरोध:"(Yogah Chitta vritti nirodhah)(Controlling of mind).

As a technique for control of prana, pranayama practice will increase the stock of prana in the body. Pranayama practices have benefits of all levels for well-beings – physical, mental and spiritual.

Why This Book?

Being myself a IT-Professional, over the years, I've seen how easy it is for professionals to prioritize productivity over health. Like many, I found myself caught in the cycle of long work hours, poor posture, and constant stress. Yoga became my lifeline—a way to restore balance, manage stress, and stay energized.

"Zen at Your Desk" is my effort to share these invaluable tools with you. This book focuses exclusively on seated yoga poses and breathing exercises that you can perform anytime, anywhere, making wellness achievable even during the busiest of days.

What You'll Gain

Through this book, you'll learn to:
- Relieve common physical discomforts like back pain and neck tension.
- Cultivate mental clarity and manage workplace stress.
- Boost your energy and productivity with quick, effective yoga routines.
- Reconnect with your breath and regain a sense of calm amidst daily chaos.

Chapter 1

About yoga

What is chair yoga?

Chair yoga is an extended form of traditional yoga. This is practice while sitting on chair, this chair yoga is designed to an individual who may have mobility issues, be recovering from injuries, or feel uncomfortable performing traditional yoga on the floor.

Understanding the Benefits of Sitting Yoga:

As working professionals does not get enough time and space to do yoga so in office chair also they can do yoga and get a benefits of serenity.

1. Chair yoga is easily doable in your office, doesn't required any special setup and other accessories.
2. Remove the fatigue from office works.
3. Helps alleviate symptoms of a sedentary lifestyle, such as stiffness and back pain.
4. Improve muscle strength.
5. Relief from eye stains.
6. improve posture, increase flexibility, improve balance while avoiding injury, reduces stress and also Enhances the blood flow.
7. Who can't sit down and practice yoga asana for them chair yoga is the ideal option.
8. Chair yoga allows people with physical limitations to experience the mental and physical benefits of yoga.
9. Yoga may lead to improvements in attention, memory, and decision-making skills, thereby enhancing job performance and productivity.
10. The practice of yoga is renowned for its stress-relieving and mood-enhancing effects, making it particularly relevant in the context of occupational well-being.
11. Regular practice of yoga can help alleviate symptoms of anxiety, depression, and mood disturbances by promoting emotional regulation and enhancing self-awareness. Yoga also encourages present-moment awareness and mindfulness, which can help individuals better cope with the challenges and demands of their work.

12.   The mindfulness practices inherent in yoga, such as focused attention on breath and body sensations, can help improve cognitive function and concentration. By training the mind to stay present and focused, yoga can enhance attentional control and mental clarity, leading to improved productivity and performance in the workplace.

13. Incorporating yoga into one's routine can help individuals achieve a better balance between work responsibilities and personal well-being. By carving out time for self-care and relaxation, employees can recharge and rejuvenate, ultimately leading to greater overall satisfaction and fulfilment both in and out of the workplace.

14. Yoga fosters a sense of connection and community among practitioners, which can translate to improved interpersonal relationships in the workplace. Participating in yoga classes or wellness programs with colleagues can promote camaraderie, teamwork, and mutual support, leading to a more positive and cohesive work environment.

Incorporating yoga into professional settings offers a holistic approach to promoting physical, mental, and emotional health among employees, ultimately fostering a more positive and productive workplace culture.

Important Instructions:

1. Listen to Your Body : Pay attention to how your body feels during practice and honour its limitations. Avoid pushing yourself into poses that feel uncomfortable or painful. Yoga need to practice as per individual's constitutions.

2. Breathe Mindfully: Focus on deep, steady breaths throughout your practice. Use your breath to guide your movements and cultivate a sense of calm and presence.

3. Respect Your Edge: Find a balance between effort and ease in each pose. Challenge yourself to explore your edge, but avoid pushing beyond your limits or forcing your body into positions it's not ready for.

4. Modify as Needed: Feel free to modify poses to suit your body and abilities. Use props such as blocks, straps, or bolsters to support your practice and make poses more accessible.

5. Stay Present: Bring your attention to the present moment by focusing on your breath, sensations in your body, and the rhythm of your movements. Let go of distractions and worries from the outside world.

6. Be Patient and Persistent: Yoga is a practice, not a performance. Progress may be gradual, so be patient with yourself and stay committed to your practice over time.

7. Practice Non-Judgment: Release any judgment or comparison during your practice. Each person's body is unique, and every day is different. Embrace where you are in your practice without self-criticism.

8. Stay Hydrated and Nourished: Drink plenty of water and stay hydrated. Fuel your body with nutritious foods to support your energy levels and recovery. Simple and nutritious food is ideal.

9. Have Fun and Enjoy the Journey: Approach your practice with a sense of joy, curiosity, and playfulness. Embrace the journey of self-discovery and self-care that yoga offers.

10. Medical conditions: If any health issues and medical history then need to be careful when practicing yoga.

11. Positive Attitude: Positive attitude removes tensions and provides focus and positive energies for inner transformation.

Prayers

Opening Prayer:

ॐसहनाववतु । सहनौभुनक्तु । सहवीर्यंकरवावहै । तेजस्विनावधीतमस्तुमाविद्विषावहै ।
ॐशान्तिः शान्तिः शान्तिः ॥

Om SahaNaav[au]-Avatu | SahaNau Bhunaktu | Saha Veeryam Karavaavahai | TejasviNaav[au]-Adhiitam-Astu Maa Vidvissaavahai | Om ShaantihShaantihShaantih||

Meaning:

1. Om, Together may we two Move (in our Studies, the Teacher and the Student)
2. Together may we two Relish (our Studies, the Teacher and the Student),
3. Together may we perform (our Studies) with Vigor (with deep Concentration),
4. May what has been Studied by us be filled with the Brilliance (of Understanding,

   leading to Knowledge); May it Not give rise to Hostility (due to lack of Understanding),

5. Om Peace, Peace, Peace.

Chapter 2

Seating warm up exercises(chair variations)

Neck Exercises

1. Side-to-Side Neck Stretch:
 Purpose: Stretches the sides of the neck and relieves lateral tension.

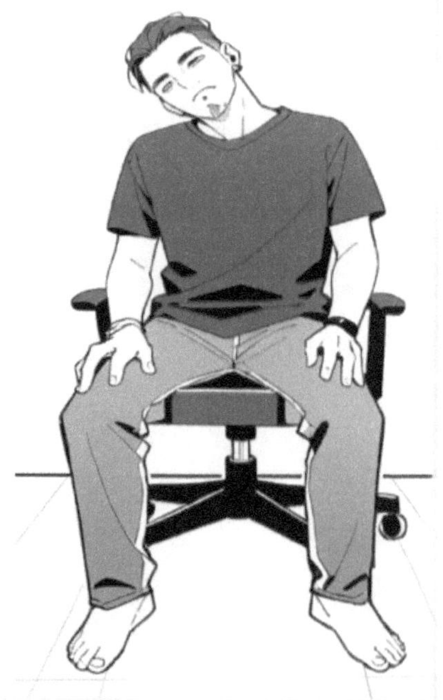

Steps:

1. Sit comfortably on chair with your back straight and shoulders relaxed.
2. Slowly tilt your head to the right, bringing your right ear toward your right shoulder.

3. Hold for 10-15 seconds and return to the centre.
4. Repeat on the left side.
5. Perform 3-5 repetitions on each side.

2. Neck Flexion and Extension

Purpose: Relieves stiffness in the front and back of the neck.

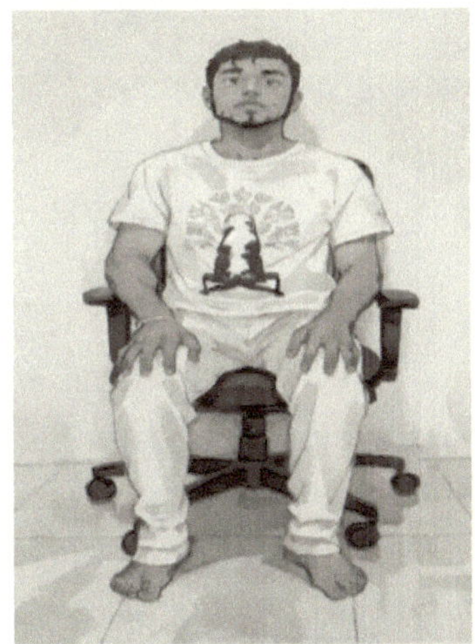

Normal   Neck Flexion

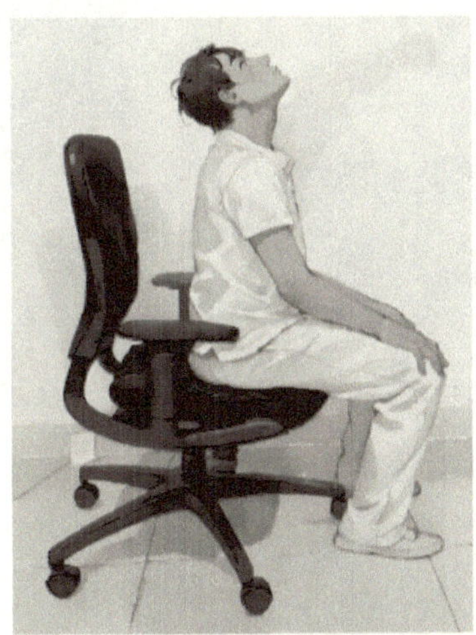

Neck Extension

Steps:

1. Sit comfortably on chair with your back straight and shoulders relaxed.
2. Slowly drop your chin toward your chest (neck flexion).
3. Hold for 5-10 seconds, then lift your head and look upward (neck extension).
4. Hold for 5-10 seconds and return to a neutral position.
5. Repeat 5-8 times.

3. Forward and Backward Neck Glide

Purpose: Strengthens neck muscles and improves posture.

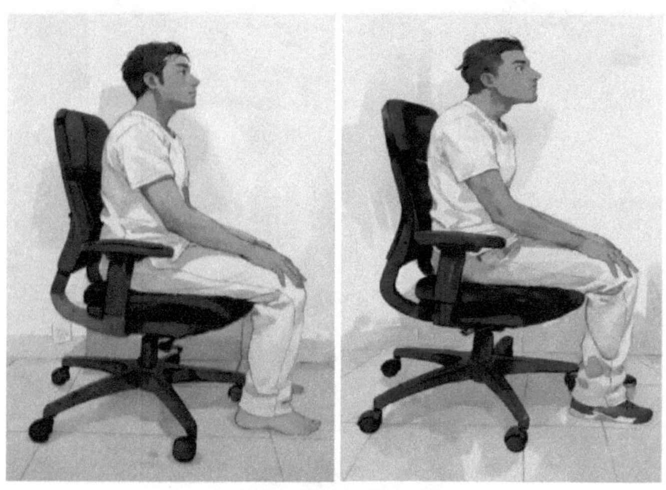

Normal   Forward Neck Glide

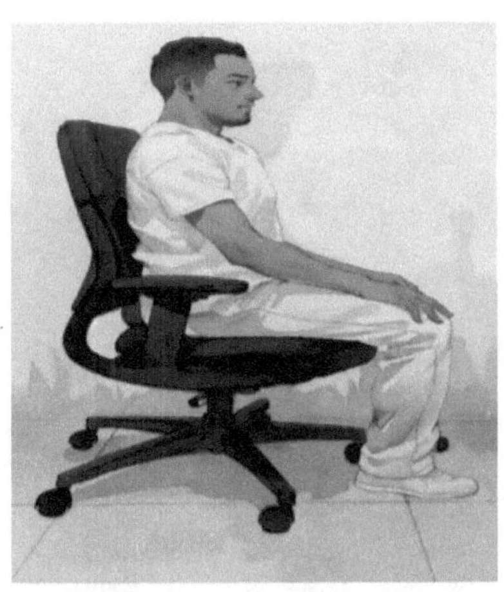

Backward Neck Glide

Steps:

a. Sit comfortably on chair with your back straight and shoulders relaxed.
b. Gently glide your head forward, jutting your chin out.
c. Glide your head backward, bringing your chin toward your neck (like making a double chin).
d. Keep the movement slow and controlled.
e. Repeat 10-12 times.

4. Neck Rotations

Purpose: Improves neck mobility and reduces stiffness from prolonged desk work.

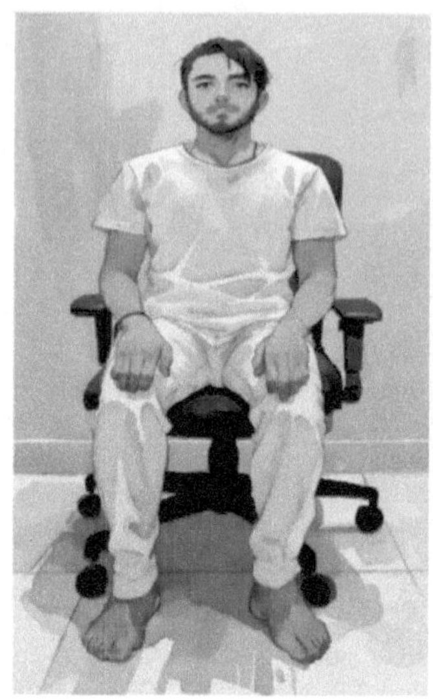 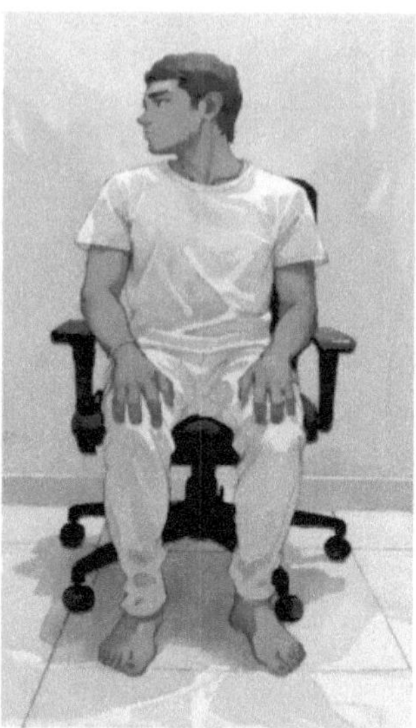

Steps:

1. Sit comfortably on chair with your back straight and shoulders relaxed.
2. Slowly turn your head to the right, looking over your shoulder.
3. Hold for 5-10 seconds, then return to the center.
4. Repeat on the left side.
5. Perform 5-8 repetitions on each side.

5. Neck Rolls

Purpose: Relieves overall neck tension and improves flexibility.

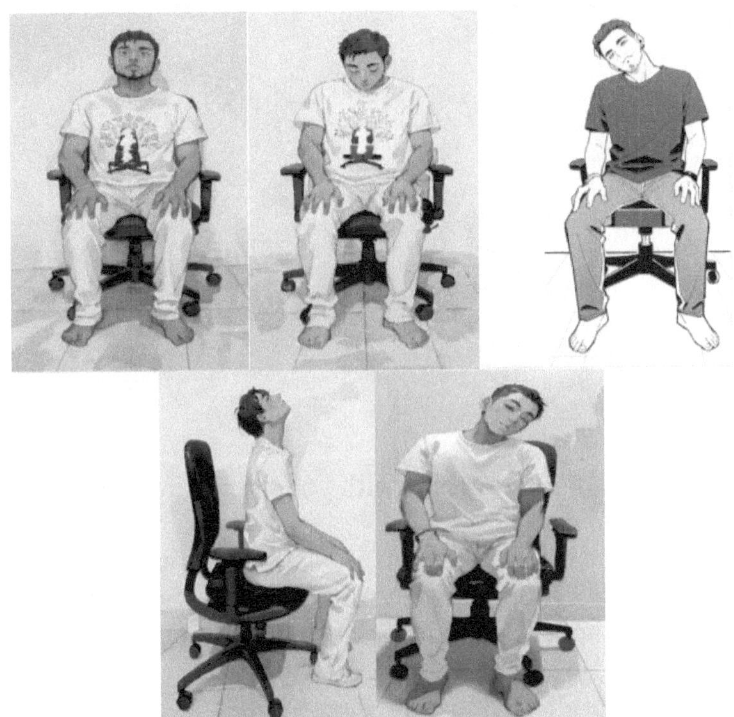

Steps:

1. Sit comfortably on chair with your back straight and shoulders relaxed.
2. Slowly drop your chin toward your chest.
3. Gently roll your head to the right, bringing your right ear toward your right shoulder.
4. Continue the roll to the back, then to the left, and back to the front.
5. Perform 3-5 slow circles clockwise, then reverse direction.

6. Upper Trapezius Stretch

Purpose: Relieves tension in the upper shoulders and sides of
the neck.

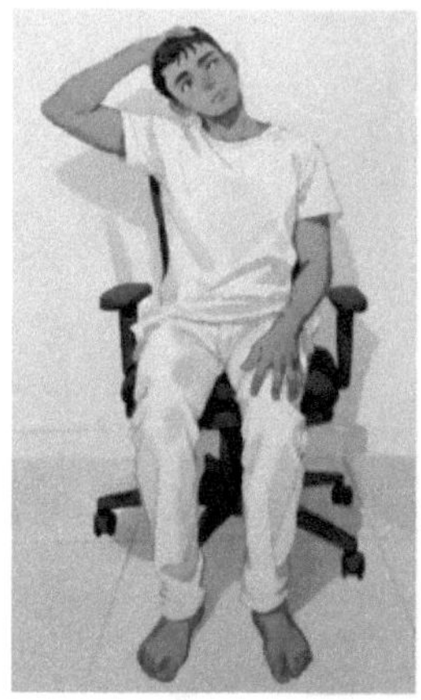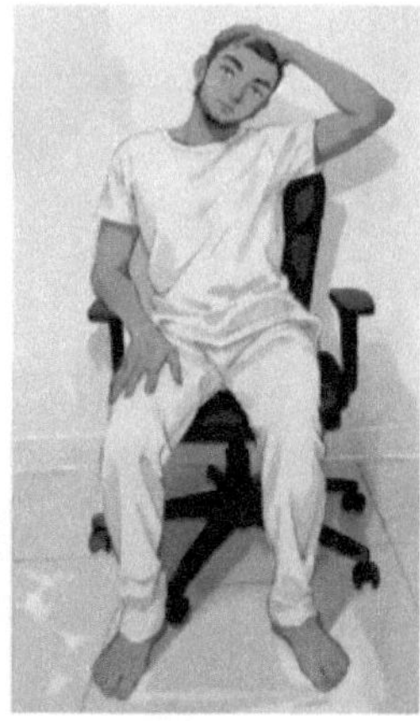

Steps:
1. Sit comfortably on chair with your back straight and
    shoulders relaxed.
2. Place your right hand on the left side of your head.
3. Gently pull your head toward your right shoulder while
    keeping the left shoulder relaxed.
4. Hold for 10-15 seconds, then switch sides.
5. Perform 3-5 repetitions on each side.

7. Chin Tucks

Purpose: Strengthens deep neck muscles and corrects forward head
posture.

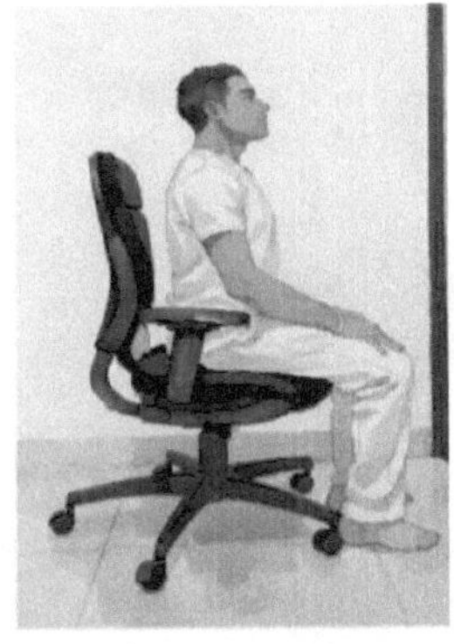 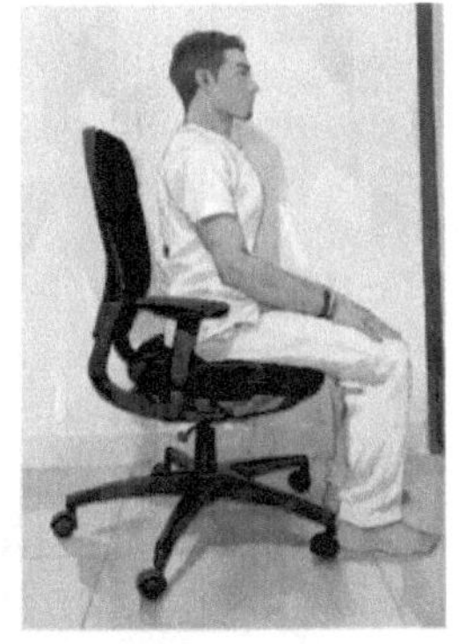

Normal head straight   Chin Tuck

Steps:

1. Sit comfortably on chair with your back straight and shoulders relaxed.
2. Tuck your chin slightly, as if trying to create a double chin.
3. Hold for 5-10 seconds and release.
4. Repeat 8-10 times.

8. Levator Scapulae Stretch

Purpose: Targets the back of the neck and upper shoulder muscles.

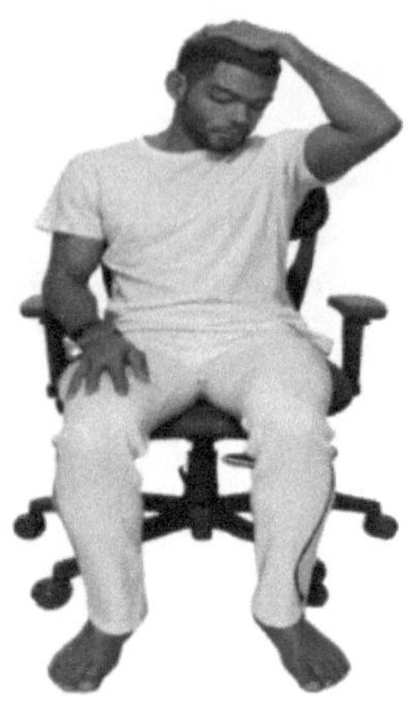

Steps:

1. Sit comfortably on chair with your back straight and shoulders relaxed.
2. Tilt your head slightly downward toward your left armpit.
3. Use your left hand to gently guide to pull your head further downward (toward the left armpit) for deeper into the stretch. But not a painful pull. Right hand can be kept down back or bring your arm up and place your hand on the back of your shoulder blade so your elbow is pointing upward
4. Hold for 10-15 seconds and switch sides.
5. Perform 3-5 repetitions on each side.

9. Shoulder Shrugs

Purpose: Relieves tension in the shoulders and neck.

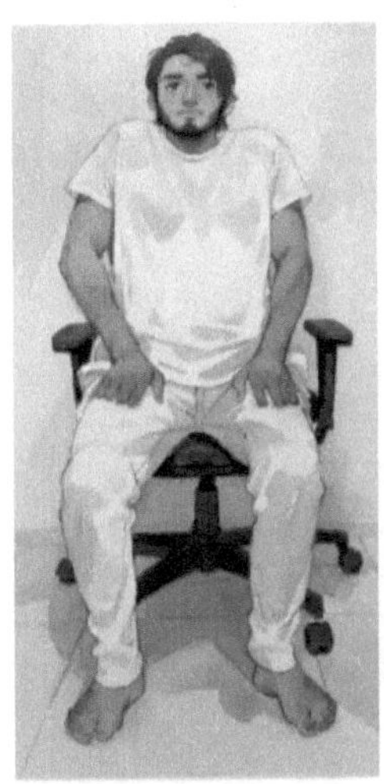

Steps:

1. Sit comfortably on chair with your back straight and shoulders relaxed.
2. Inhale and lift your shoulders toward your ears.
3. Hold for 1-2 seconds, then exhale and release them down.
4. Repeat 8-10 times.

Seated Spinal Twist:

The Seated Spinal Twist is a yoga pose performed while seated on a chair or the floor, where the practitioner gently rotates the upper body to one side. It focuses on improving spinal flexibility, releasing tension in the back and shoulders, and promoting better posture. This pose is particularly beneficial for desk workers, as it counteracts the stiffness caused by prolonged sitting. The seated spinal twist is an excellent stretch to relieve tension in the spine, improve posture, and enhance flexibility. It's ideal for IT professionals who spend long hours sitting at a desk.

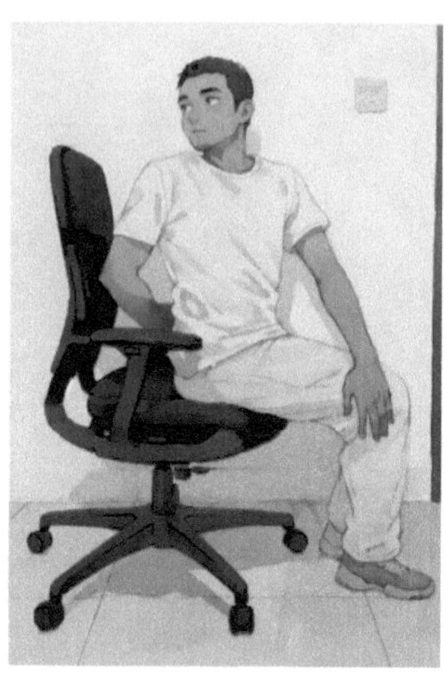

Steps to Perform:

1. Start Position:
    o Sit comfortably on a chair with your back straight and feet flat on the ground.
    o Keep your shoulders relaxed and your hands resting on your thighs.
2. Twist to the Right:
    o Place your right hand on the backrest of the chair.
    o Place your left hand on the outside of your right thigh.
    o Inhale deeply, lengthening your spine as you sit up tall.
3. Deepen the Stretch:
    o Exhale and gently twist your torso to the right, turning your head to look over your right shoulder.
    o Keep your hips and legs steady, allowing the twist to come from your spine and upper body.
4. Hold the Pose:
    o Hold the twist for 10-15 seconds while breathing deeply and steadily.
    o With each exhale, try to deepen the twist slightly, without forcing.

5. Return to Center:
    o Inhale and slowly untwist, returning to the neutral
       seated position.
6. Twist to the Left:
    o Repeat the same steps on the left side, placing your
       left hand on the backrest and your right hand on the
       outside of your left thigh.
7. Repetition:
    o Perform 2-3 twists on each side for maximum
       benefit.

Benefits:

- Relieves lower back and mid-back tension.
- Improves spinal mobility and flexibility.
- Promotes better posture by releasing tight muscles.
- Enhances blood circulation in the spine and surrounding
  muscles.

Hand Exercises:

Hand exercises are designed to relieve tension, improve flexibility,
and prevent repetitive strain injuries (RSI) like carpal tunnel
syndrome, which are common among IT professionals due to
prolonged typing and mouse usage.

Process 1.

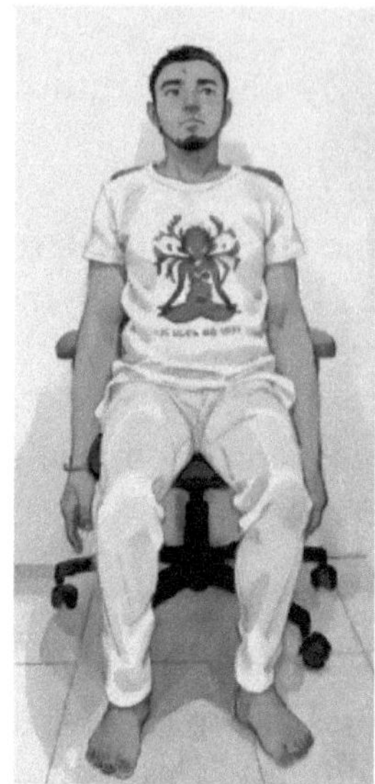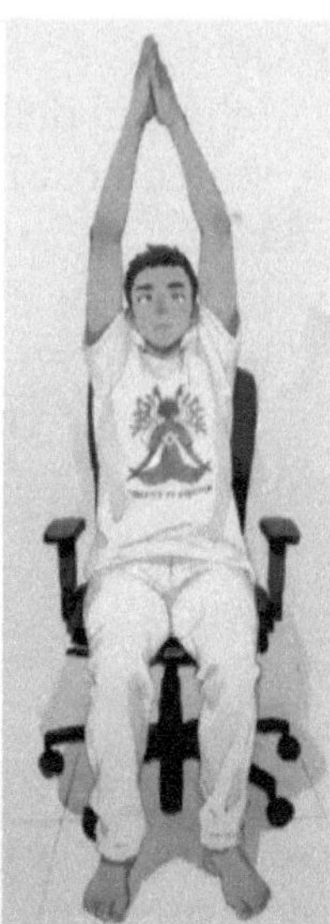

Steps:

1. Sit comfortably on a chair with your back straight and feet flat on the ground.
2. Keep your hands sidewise relaxed downwards.
3. Lift your hands above the head to the full stretch and joins the palms and fingers together. The arms should be close to the ears. Keep up in the position for 10 seconds.
4. Then bring the arms down to the earlier starting position and rest for 2 normal breaths.

Posture 2:

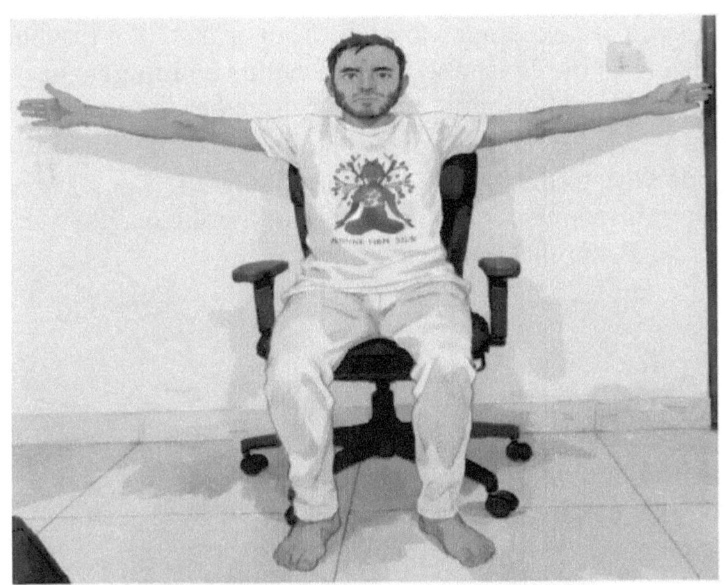

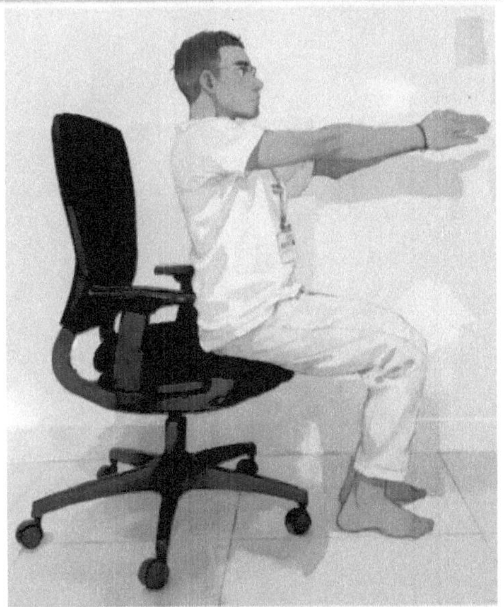

Steps:

1. Sit comfortably on a chair with your back straight and feet flat on the ground.
2. Spread the hands sideways at the shoulder level let the palms face in front.

3. As you are exhaling Move the both arms to the front at 90 degree to the chest and join the palms and fingers in front of the chest and bringing the hands together.
4. As you are inhaling, Spread the hands by moving them sideways to the back at the shoulder level.
5. Do this exercise 5/10 times by moving the hands front and back. Bring the arms down.

Wrist Flexor Stretch:

Purpose: Relieves tension in the wrists and forearms. Can also helps to relieve pain and stiffness in the wrist by loosening up tight muscles.

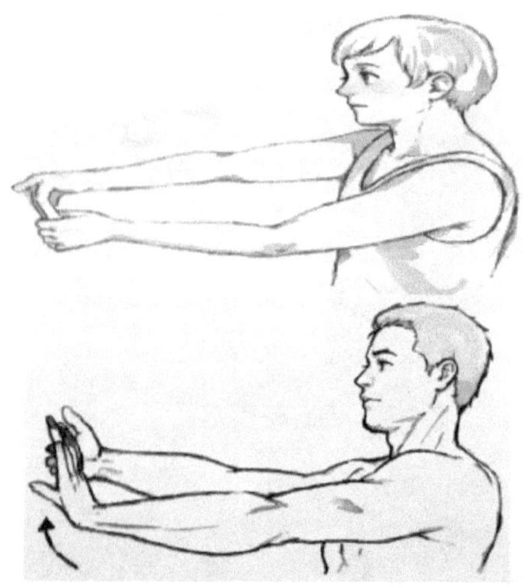

Steps:

o Sit comfortably with your back straight Sit comfortably with your back straight on chair and feet flat on the ground.
o Extend your right arm forward, palm facing up.
o Use your left hand to gently press the fingers of your right hand back toward your body.
o Hold for 10-15 seconds and switch sides.

Wrist Extensor Stretch:

Purpose: Loosens the top of the wrist and forearm.

Steps:

- Extend your right arm forward, palm facing down.
- Use your left hand to press the fingers of your right hand downward.
- Hold for 10-15 seconds and switch sides.

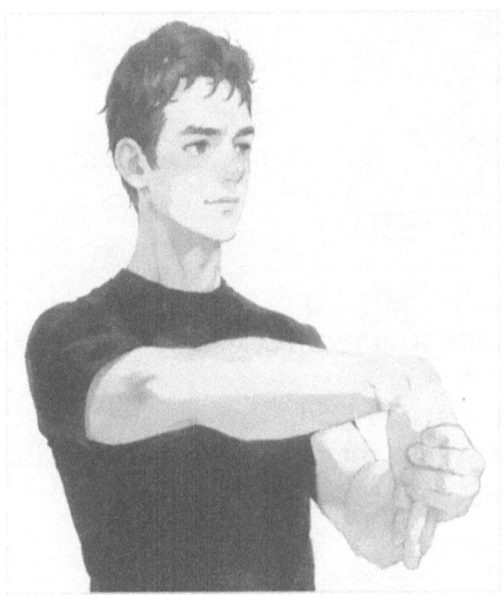

Wrist Rotate:

Purpose: Improves wrist mobility and circulation. Release the wrist pain.

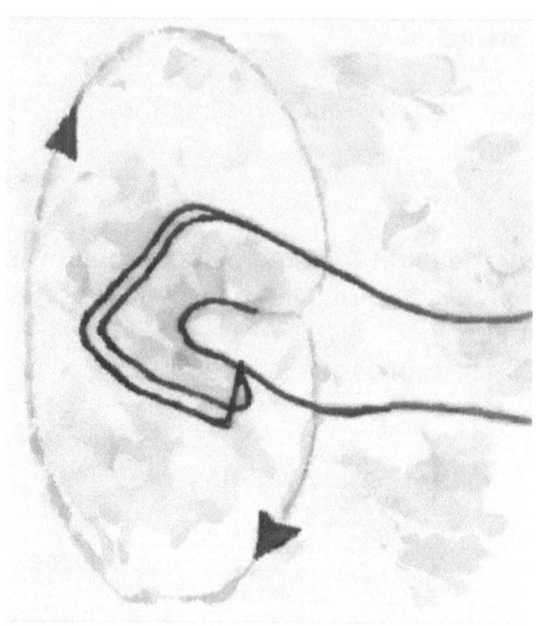

Steps:

- Sit comfortably with your back straight on chair and feet flat on the ground.
- Extend your arms forward.
- Make a fist(मुट्ठी) and rotate your wrists clockwise for 10 times.
- And anti clockwise for another 10 times.

Shoulder Exercises:

These shoulder exercises help reduce tension, improve posture, and prevent stiffness caused and increase flexibility by prolonged desk work.

1. **Shoulder Rolls:** Relieves tension in the upper shoulders and neck.

Steps:

o   Sit comfortably with your back straight on chair and feet flat on the ground.
o   Lift your shoulders toward ears.
o   Roll them backward in a circular motion for 10 round.
o   Repeat the motion forward for another 10 round.

2. **Shoulder Shrugs:** Reduces muscle tightness in the trapezius area.

Steps:
o   On chair, sit upright with feet flat on the floor and relax your arms at your sides.
o   Lift both shoulders up towards ears.
o   Hold for 3-5 seconds and then relax.
o   Repeat 8-10 times.

3. **Shoulder Squeeze Exercise:** Improves posture and relieves pain, tension in the mid-back and shoulders.

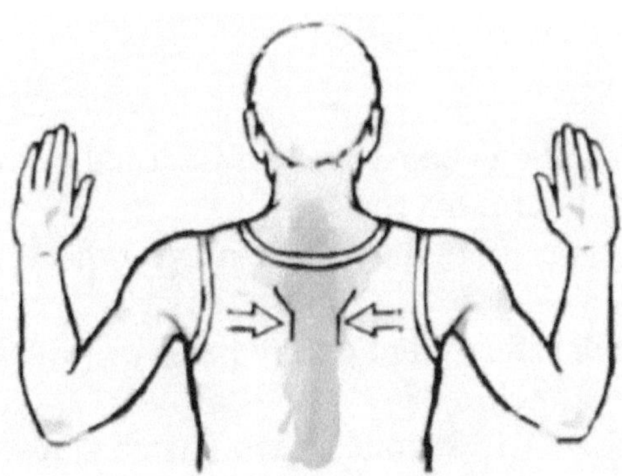

Steps:

1.   Sit upright on chair with feet flat on the floor.

2. Bring your arms to shoulder height, bending elbows at 90 degrees.
3. Squeeze your shoulder blades together as if trying to hold a pencil between them.
4. Hold for 5 seconds and release.
5. Repeat 8-10 times.

4. Overhead Shoulder Stretch: Stretches the sides of the shoulders and upper back.

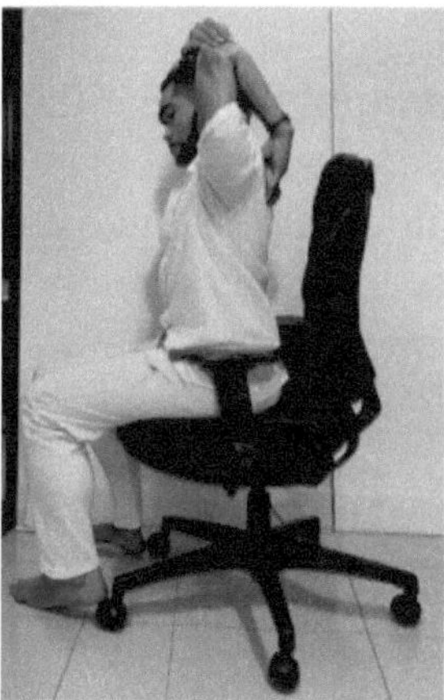

Steps:

- Sit upright on chair with feet flat on the floor and extend your right arm overhead.
- Bend your right elbow, placing your hand between your shoulder blades.
- Use your left hand to gently press on your right elbow for a deeper stretch.
- Hold for 10-15 seconds, then switch sides.

6. **Arm Circles:** Enhances shoulder mobility and improves circulation.

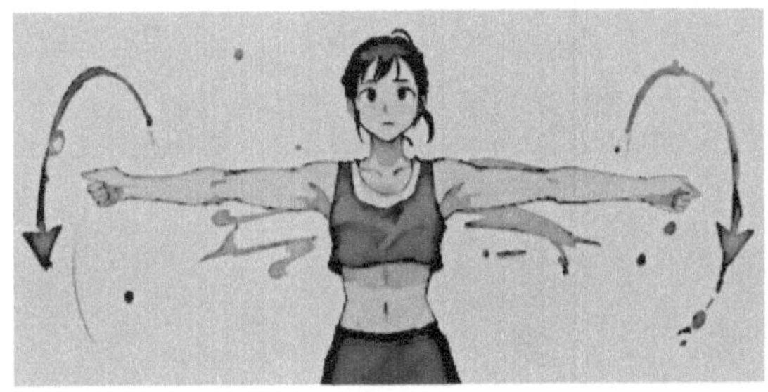

Steps:

- o   Stand or sit with arms extended to the sides.
- o   Make small circles with your arms for 10 seconds.
- o   Gradually make larger circles for another 10 seconds.
- o   Reverse the direction(first clock and then anti clockwise) and repeat.

7. **Cross-Body Shoulder Stretch:**
   Stretches the back of the shoulder and deltoids.

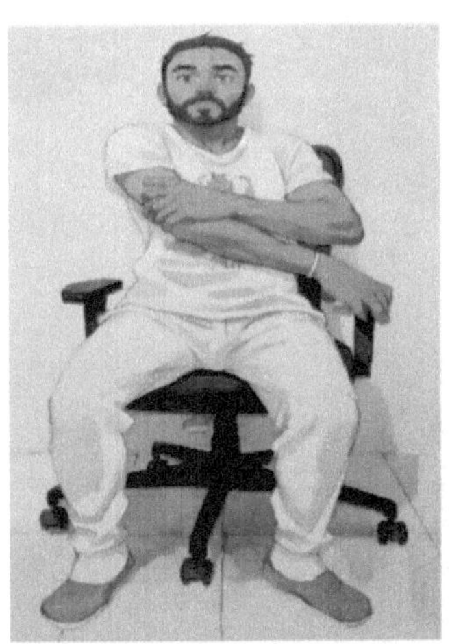

Steps:

- o Extend your right arm across your chest.
- o Use your left hand to gently press the right arm closer to your chest.
- o Hold for 10-15 seconds, then switch sides.

Leg Exercises

6. Leg Lifts and strait:

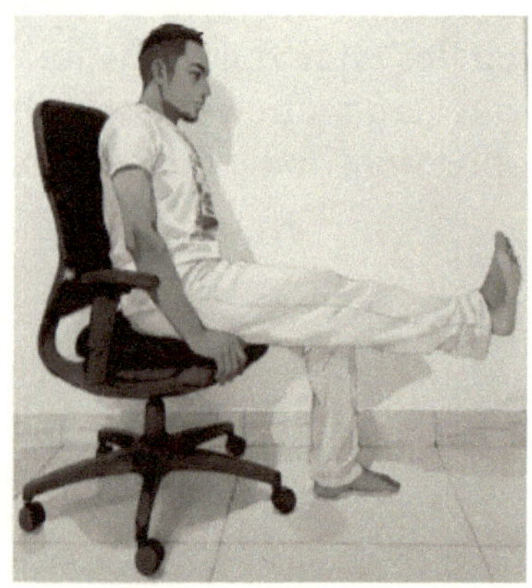

Steps:

- o Sit on chair keeping your back straight.
- o Keep your feet flat on the floor and knees bent at 90 degrees.
- o Slowly extend and lift your right leg until it is parallel to the floor.
- o Hold for 5 seconds, then lower it back down.
- o Repeat with same with left leg.
- o Repeat the process for 10–12 times per leg.

7. Heel-to-Toe Taps(Up & Down):

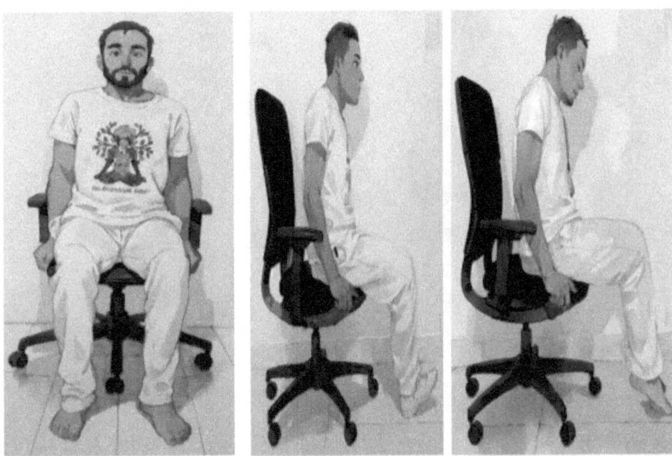

Steps:

- o   Keep your feet flat on the floor.
- o   Lift your toes up while keeping your heels on the floor.
- o   Lower your toes and lift your heels up instead.
- o   Alternate between the two.
- o   Repeat the process for 20 to 25 taps.

8.   Seated Marching Stretch:

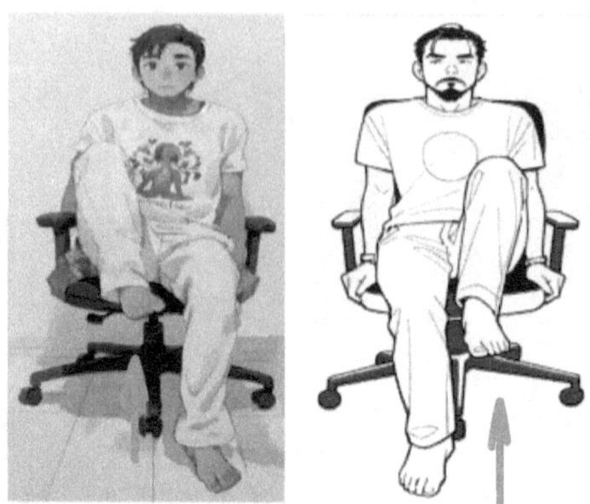

Steps:

- o Sit in chair upright and keep your feet flat on the floor.
- o Slowly lift right knee as high as you can towards your chest, then lower your foot to the floor.
- o Then practice the same with your left knee.
- o Continue alternating in a marching motion.
- o Repeat this for 60 seconds.

9. Ankle movement (Forwards and Backwards):

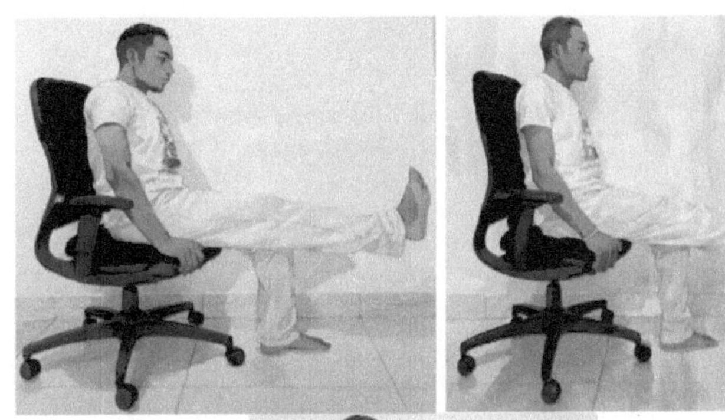

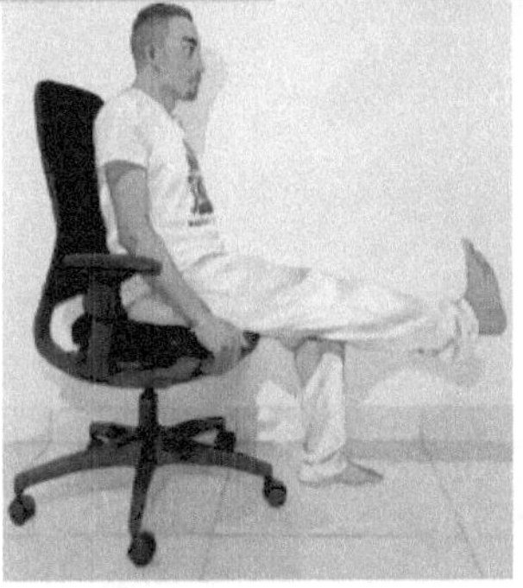

Steps:
- o Sit in chair upright and keep your feet flat on the floor.
- o Slowly lift your right leg off the ground and make knee straight and move the feet forward and backward. Do it for 20 times.
- o Then practice it for left leg as well.
- o Repeat the practice 30 to 60 seconds.

10. Ankle Rotations:

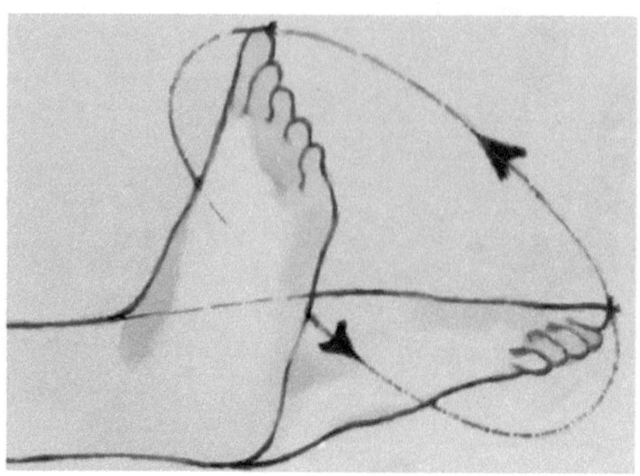

Steps:

- Sit in chair upright with your feet flat on the floor.
- Lift your right foot slightly off the ground and make knee straight .
- Rotate your ankle clockwise for 5–10 seconds, then anti-clockwise.
- Switch to the left foot and repeat the same process.
- 5/10 rotations per direction for each foot.

11. Seated Calf Raise:

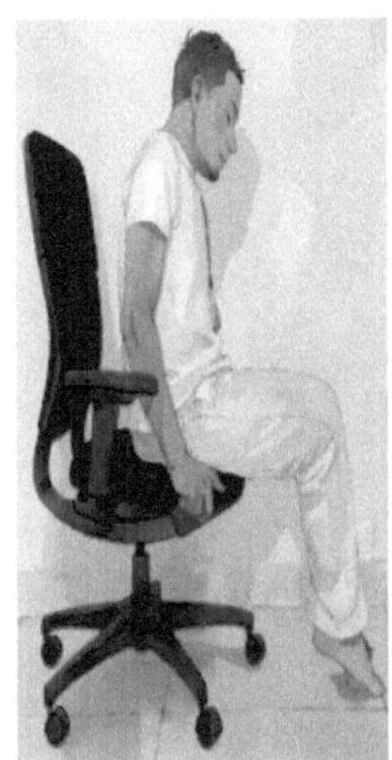

Steps:
- Sit in chair with your feet flat on the ground.
- Raise your heels off the floor as high as possible, keeping your toes planted on ground.
- Slowly lower your heels back down.
- Repeats the same for 12 to 15 times or as long as you like when you are working and seated in chair.

12. Seated-Leg Circles:

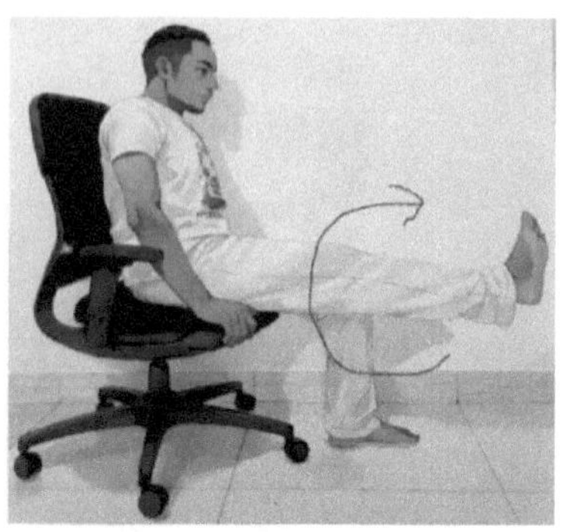

Steps:
- o   Sit in chair and maintain good posture.
- o   Extend your right leg out straight off the floor.
- o   Make small circular motions in the air with your foot.
- o   Perform 10 clockwise and 10 anticlockwise circles.
- o   Switch to the left leg.

13. Seated Knee Flexion & Extensions:

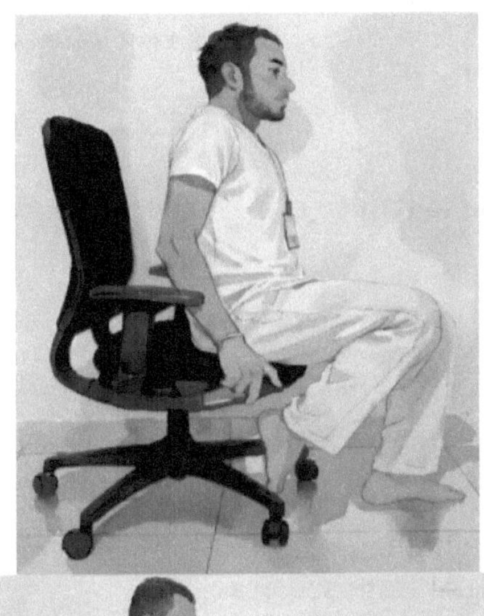

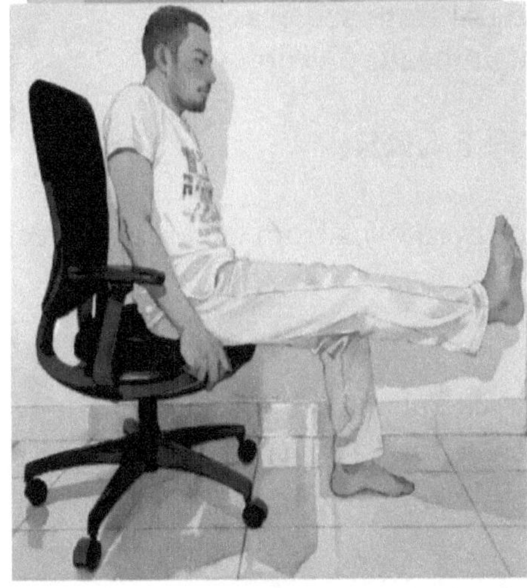

Steps:
- Sit upright and hold the sides of the chair for balance.
- Take your right knee as far back as possible hold for few seconds and Extend your right leg straight out in front of you and hold for at least 10 seconds.
- Slowly bend it back to the starting position.
- Repeat with the same with left leg.

o   Repeat the process for 10 to 15 times for each leg.

Eye Exercises

1. 20-20-20 Rule

Simple technique to reduce eye fatigue while working or traveling.

Process:

Every 20 minutes, look at an object 20 feet away for 20 seconds.

Benefits:

1. Prevents eye strain
2. Reduces fatigue from screens
3. Helps maintain healthy vision

2. Blinking Eye Exercise

Useful for dry or tired eyes from excessive screen time.

Process:

1. Keep your eyes open and blink rapidly for 15 seconds.
2. Close your eyes for 15 seconds and relax.
3. Repeat 3–5 times.

Benefits:

1. Lubricates the eyes.
2. Improves eye muscle coordination.
3. Reduces eye dryness.

3. Eye Rolling (Clockwise & Anti-Clockwise)

Strengthens eye muscles and improves flexibility.

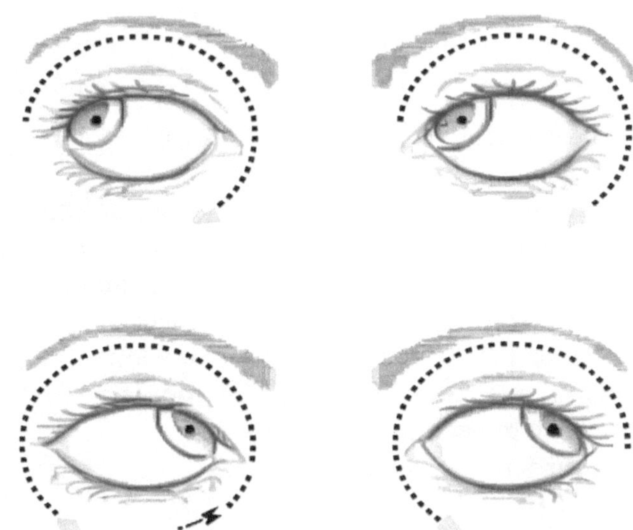

Process:

1. Sit comfortably in chair and look straight ahead.
2. Slowly move your eyes clockwise in a circular motion.
3. Repeat 5 times, then switch to anti-clockwise.
4. Close your eyes to relax.

Benefits:

1. Enhances eye muscle flexibility.
2. Helps with eye strain and fatigue.
3. Improves blood circulation.

4. Eye Movement

Horizontal Movement:

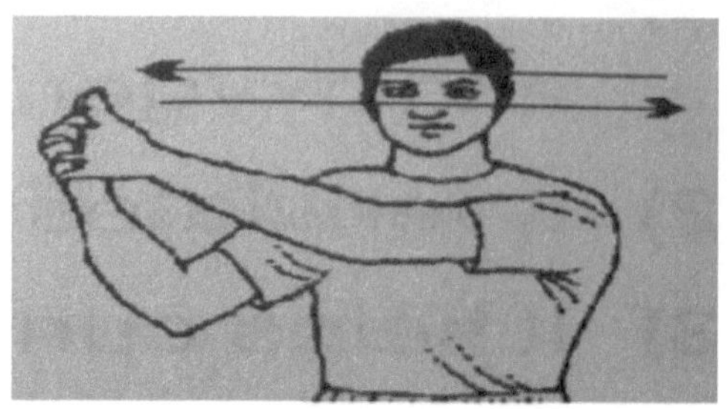

Process:

1. Sit in chair with your feet flat on the ground.
2. Maintain spine straight.
3. Now clasp hands with the thumbs together upright. Raise the clasped hands to a level slightly lower than the eyes and keep elbows slightly bent. Focus the top on the thumb-nails. Keep this posture throughout these eye exercise.
4. Move the hands horizontally to right and left extreme. The eyes should move along with the thumbs from left to extreme right and from there back to the extreme left.
5. Do this for 5 times.

Vertical Eye Movement:

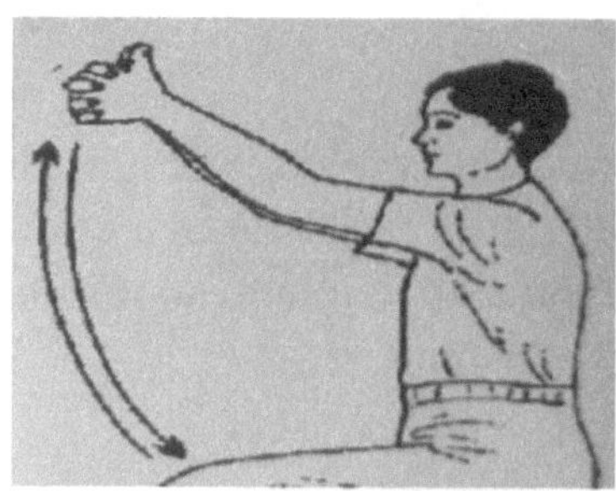

Process:

1. Now with the eyes fixed on the thumbnails, keep your hands on your lap near the knees.
2. Lift the hands vertically upwards as far as possible and bring them down to the lap, swinging the eyes up and down along

with the thumbs. Only the eyes should move with up-and-down movement of hands.
3. Do this exercise 5 times.

Diagonal Movement:

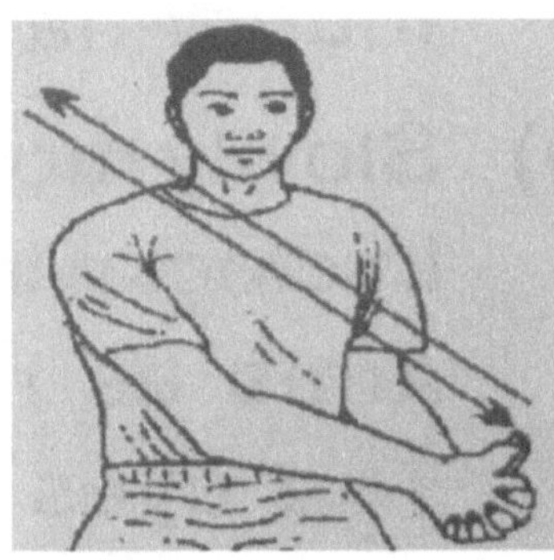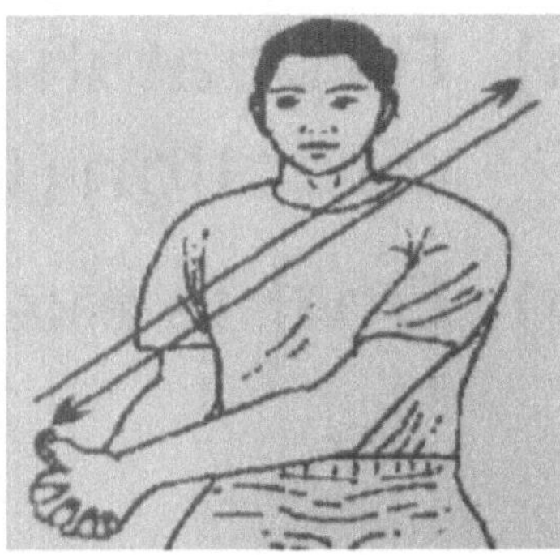

Process:

1. Now keep your hands with thumbs together upright near the outside of your left thigh.
2. Move the hands up and down diagonally starting from left lower corner (thigh) to right upper corner(shoulder).
3. Same way other side diagonally, from right thigh to upper left corner shoulder.
4. Repeat both side 5, 5 times.

Benefits:

1. Strengthens Eye Muscles.
2. Improves Eye Coordination & Focus.
3. Reduces Digital Eye Strain.
4. Enhances Brain Function & Concentration.

5. Palming (Warmth & Relaxation)

Great for instant relaxation and reducing eye fatigue.

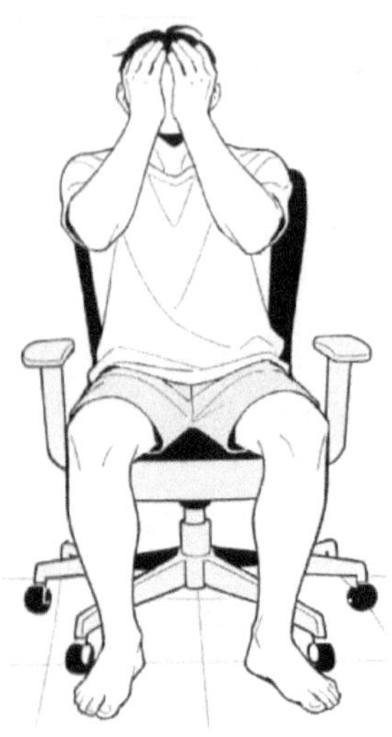

Process:

1. Rub your palms together briskly until they feel warm.
2. Close your eyes and cup your palms over them without pressing. Left eye with left palm and right eye with right palm.
3. Breathe deeply and relax for 30–60 seconds.
   Repeat for about 5 times.

Benefits:

1. Relaxes the optic nerve.
2. Reduces stress and strain.
3. Helps relieve headaches.

Chapter 3

Seated Asana-Chair variations

<h1 style="text-align:center">Seated Asana</h1>

These seated yoga poses are specifically designed for Software and other professionals to alleviate stress, improve posture, and enhance flexibility, while sitting on a chair. These asanas can be performed during short breaks without needing additional equipment considering stomach is empty enough for asana.

Seated Trikonasana(Trianlge chair pose):

'Tri' means three and 'Kona' means 'corner'. So, trikonasana literally translates to 'Three-corners'. It is named so as the final posture resembles a triangle formed by the torso, upper limbs and lower limbs. Chair Variant for working engineers should be adapted to suit long sitting hours, focusing on spinal mobility, lateral stretching, and ease of practice at a workstation.

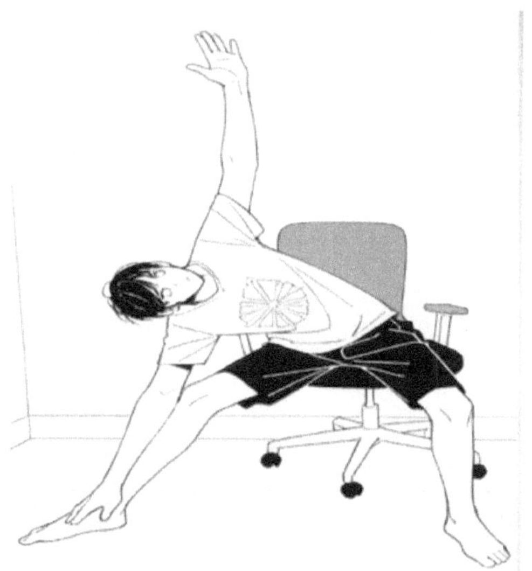

Steps to practice:

1. Sit sideways on the chair with your feet flat on the floor and your spine upright.

2. If your chair has armrests, ensure they don't restrict your movement.
3. Extend one right leg straight out to the side while keeping the left leg bent at a 90-degree angle with the foot grounded. Both feet should firmly planted to maintain stability.
4. Inhale and extend both arms outward at shoulder level.
5. Exhale and bend sideways towards the extended right leg, placing the lower hand on the shin, ankle.
6. The top arm reaches upward, in line with the shoulders, while you look at your raised hand or keep your head neutral.
7. Keep your chest open and engage your core.
8. Hold the pose for 15 seconds.
9. Inhale to come back to the center and switch to other sides.

Benefits:

1. Stretches and opens the hips, groins, hamstrings, calves, shoulders, chest and spine.
2. Increases mental and physical equilibrium. Enhances focus and relieves stiffness from prolonged sitting.
3. Helps improve digestion.
4. Reduces anxiety, stress, back pain and sciatica.
5. Improves lateral flexibility and posture.

🚫 Contraindications:

Avoid if you have below issues

1. Severe spinal disorders, herniated discs, or recent surgery.
2. Individuals with high blood pressure or dizziness should practice with caution.
3. If you experience discomfort, modify by keeping the twist gently.

Seated Parivartta Trikonasana (Chair pose):

In Sanskrit, 'parivrtta' means revolved; 'trikona' means triangle, and 'asana' means posture. Parivrtta trikonasana is a standing plus twisting yogasana that is regarded as a perfect balancing pose. Chair Variant for working engineers should be adapted to suit long sitting hours, focusing on spinal mobility, lateral stretching, and ease of practice at a workstation.

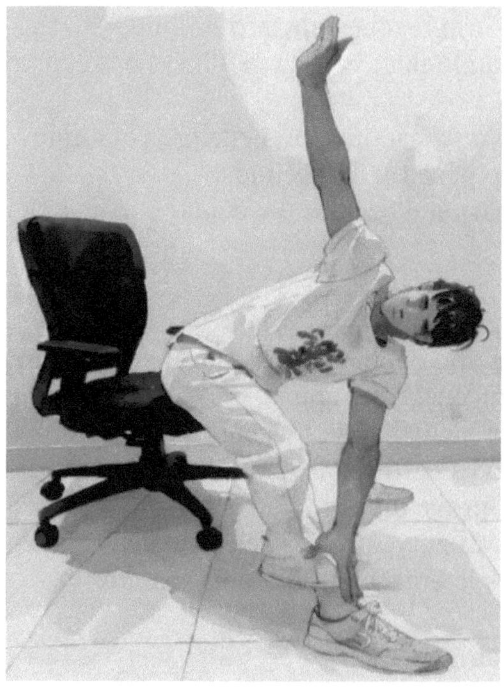

Steps to practice:

1. Sit sideways on a sturdy chair with your feet flat on the floor.
2. Keep your knees bent at 90 degrees and your spine upright.
3. Extend your right leg sideways, keeping it straight, with your toes pointing forward.
4. Keep your left foot flat on the floor, maintaining stability.
5. Twisting the Torso and Place your left hand on the outside of your right ankle if not flexible then you can touch knee.

6. Inhale deeply, lengthen your spine, and as you exhale, twist your torso toward the right.
7. Raise your right arm straight up, aligning it with your shoulder.
8. Gaze upward toward your raised hand or keep your neck in a neutral position.
9. Hold for 15 second.
10. Inhale and slowly come back.
11. Bring your right leg back and sit facing forward.
12. Repeat the pose on the other side.

Benefits:

Parivrtta trikonasana will squeeze the abdominal organs, creating a wringing action so that when released, a fresh supply of blood will be flushed into these vital organs. As a result,

1. Thigh, calf and hamstring muscles get toned.
2. The spine and back muscles work better. Improves posture and relieves stiffness from prolonged sitting.
3. There is relief from back pain. Stretches and strengthens the back, shoulders, and legs.
4. Abdominal organs are invigorated, and hip muscles are strengthened.
5. Reduces neck and shoulder tension caused by long screen time.
6. It is recommended for persons suffering from sciatica, asthma, and digestive problems including constipation.

🚫 Contraindications:

Avoid if you have below issues

1. Severe spinal disorders, herniated discs, or recent surgery.
2. Individuals with high blood pressure or dizziness should practice with caution.
3. If you experience discomfort, modify by keeping the twist gently.

Seated Garudhasana-Chair variation:

It's a standing balance asana. Garudha is mythical Bird, the bahana of Vishnu. The chair variation can be very use full for the working professional who spend long hours at a desk. It helps to relax the shoulders, stretch the upper back, and improve focus while being accessible in a seated position. This can be easily done at your desk without moving away from your work station.

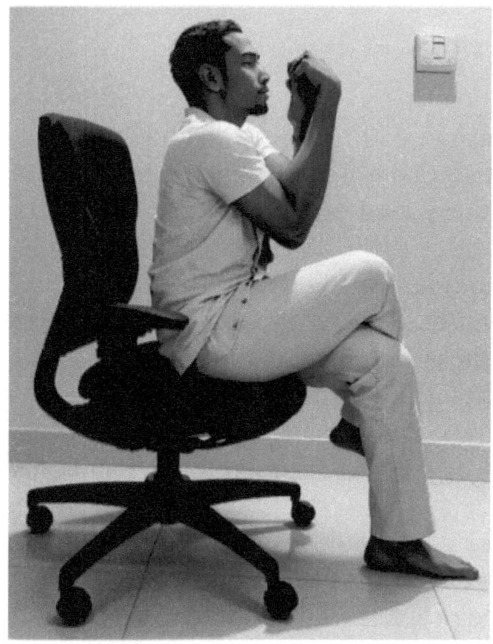

Steps:

1. Sit comfortably on a chair with your feet flat on the floor and your spine straight.
2. Keep your knees bent at 90 or 110 degrees and shoulders relaxed.
3. Cross your right thigh over your left thigh.
4. If flexibility allow you then you can hook your right foot behind your left calf.

5. If not, simply keep the right foot resting on the floor or over the left shin.
6. Extend both arms in front of you at shoulder height.
7. Cross your left arm over the right so that the elbows stack.
8. Bend your elbows, bringing the forearms perpendicular to the ground.
9. If possible, wrap your forearms around each other so that the palms touch.
10. Keep your shoulders down and away from your ears.
11. Hold the pose for 15 seconds, breathing deeply and feeling the stretch in your shoulders and upper back.
12. Inhale and slowly unwind your arms and legs.
13. Return to a neutral seated position.
14. Repeat the pose on the opposite side (left leg over right, right arm over left).

Benefits:

1. Stretches the shoulders, elbows, wrists, and upper back when seated at a desk for long hours.
2. Improves focus & concentration, making it a great mid-work break.
3. Stretches the upper back, arms, and hips, improving flexibility.
4. Enhances circulation in the legs, preventing stiffness from sitting too long.
5. Helps maintain good posture by engaging core muscles.

🚫 Contraindications:

Don't practice if you have below issues

1. Having severe shoulder, knee, or hip injuries.
2. If experiencing pain or discomfort, modify the pose by keeping your feet on the floor.
3. If with high blood pressure or vertigo should practice with caution.

Seated Ardhakati Chakrasan(Chair variation):

The Seated Ardhakati Chakrasan-Chair Variation is a modified version of the traditional Ardhakati Chakrasan (Half Wheel pose), performed while sitting on a chair for working professional. This variation allows you to experience the benefits of the posture without requiring you to get on the floor with yoga mat, making it perfect for office workers or those with limited mobility and time.

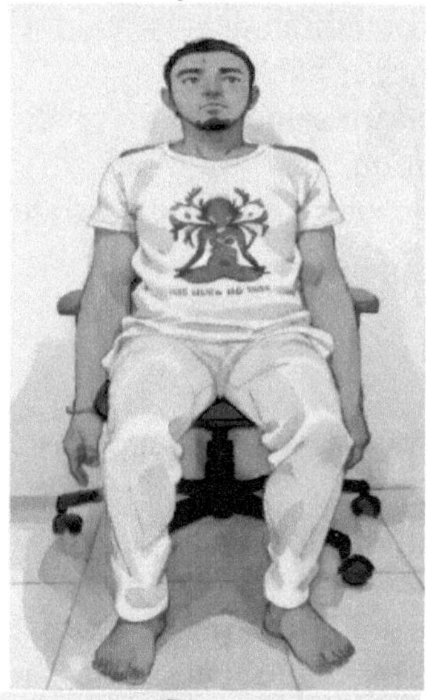

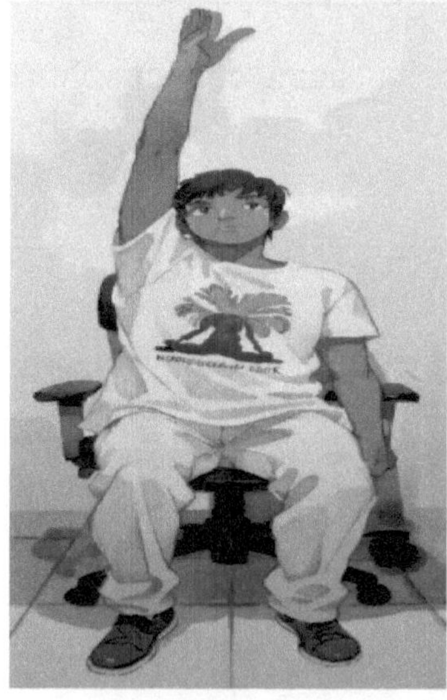

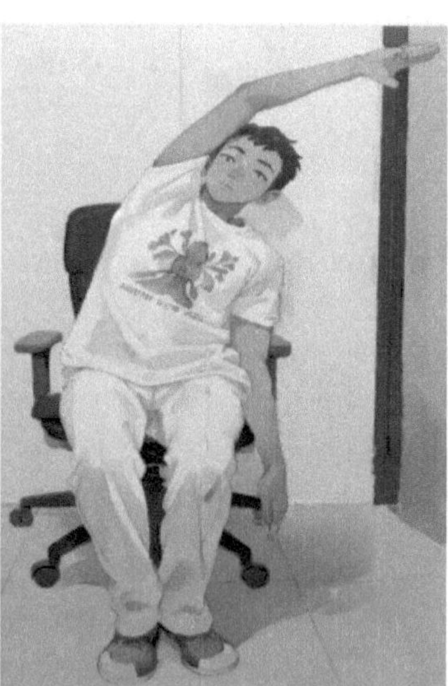

Steps:
1. Sit on the Chair: Sit upright on a chair with your feet flat on the floor and your knees bent at 90 degrees. Keep your back straight, shoulders relaxed, and hands resting on your thighs or the sides of the chair.

2. While inhaling, Raise your right arm straight up towards the ceiling, keeping your elbow straight.
3. Now while exhaling, slowly bend your trunk towards left side reach your right hand over your head to the left side, create like a half circle and feeling a gentle stretch along the right side of your torso. You can keep your left hand resting on the chair or on your left thigh for support.

4. Stay in this position for 30-60 seconds, breathing deeply and ensuring your body is aligned. Try to maintain an open chest as you stretches.

5. While inhaling, bring your right arm back to the center, returning to the starting position.

6. Repeat on the same with Other Side: Repeat the same process on the left side by raising your left arm up, reaching it over to the right, and holding the stretch.

Benefits:
1. Stretches and opens the side body, particularly the intercostal muscles, which can help with deep breathing and relaxation.
2. Improves flexibility in the spine and shoulders.
3. Reduces fat in waist region, stimulates sides of the body.
4. Gives lateral bending to the spine, improves function of liver. Relieves tension from the neck and back, making it a great option for office workers.

🚫 Contraindications:

Any individual should take precautions when they suffer from severe back pain neck pain, Shoulder and spine injuries. Recent Abdominal Surgery. Any medical condition, take professional advice before practicing.

Seated Spine twist(Chair variation):

Seated Spine twist's sanskrit name is Parivrtta Sukhasana. It's Chair Variation can be easily achieved by working professional at their desk and get the similar benefits of Parivrtta Sukhasana. It's very simple but yet very effective yoga pose.

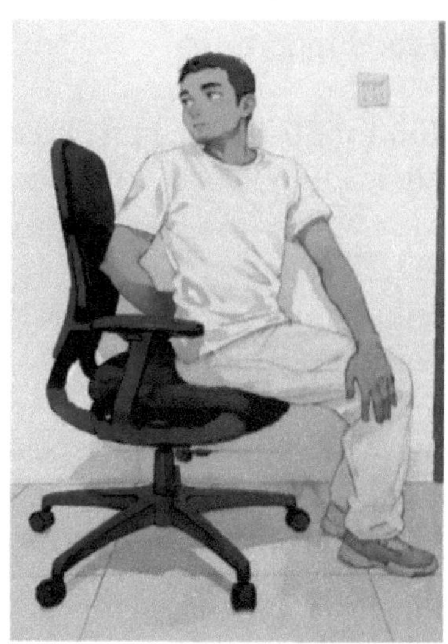

Steps:
1. Sit upright in a chair slightly forward of your chair with your feet flat on the ground, Keeping your back straight and shoulders relaxed.
2. Inhale and place your left hand on right knee and right hand of your back.
3. Exhale and gently twist your torso towards right. Avoid force twisting.
4. Keep your spine and body relaxed. Maintain the normal breathing in final posture.

5. Hold the twisting pose for 30 – 60 seconds.
6. Inhale and slowly return to the center position.
7. Now repeat the same for other side as well.

Benefits:
1. Get benefited from stress and anxiety.
2. Improves digestion.
3. Enhances flexibility in back and chest.
4. Good for diabetics.

🚫 Contraindications:

Avoid if you are having
1. spine surgery or severe back injuries.
2. Any medical condition, take professional advice before
   practicing.

Seated Tadasana(Chair variation):

Tadasana is known as mountain pose. Tadasana Chair Variation is
a modified version of Tadasana performed while sitting on a chair
at your desk. is a simple yet effective pose to improve posture,
lengthen the spine, and relieve tension, all while staying seated. It's
ideal for the working professionals.

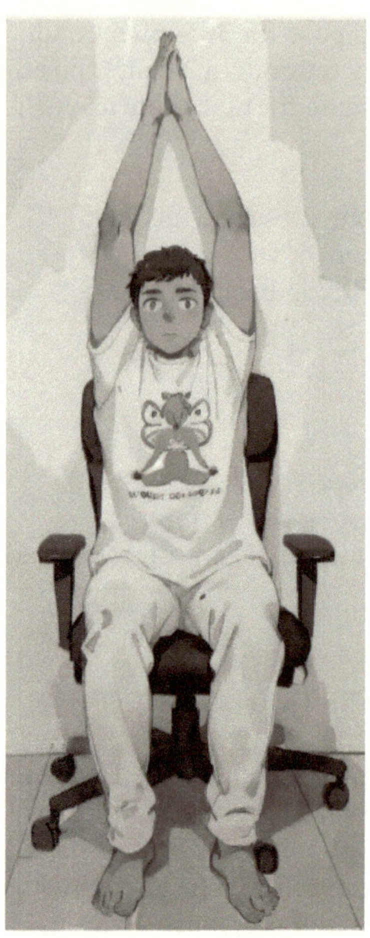

Steps:
1. Sit upright with your feet flat on the floor and knees at hip-width.
2. Keep your back straight and shoulders relaxed.
3. Inhale deeply and extend both arms overhead, keeping them shoulder-width apart.
4. Stretch your fingers upward, feeling a gentle lift in the spine.
5. Slightly pull your navel inward to activate your core muscles.
6. Avoid arching your lower back excessively.
7. Stay in the position for 30 to 60 seconds, breathing deeply.
8. Keep your neck relaxed and gaze forward or slightly upward.
9. Release the Pose and relax.

10. After inhaling as Exhaling slowly lower your arms back to the
sides.

Benefits:
1. Helps counteract slouching and spinal compression.
2. Reduces Shoulder & Neck Tension – Relieves stiffness from
    prolonged screen time.
3. Enhances Breathing Capacity – Opens the chest and lungs for
    better oxygen flow.
4. Boosts Energy & Focus – Refreshes the mind, improving
    concentration.

🚫 Contraindications:

Avoid if you are having
3. spine surgery or severe back injuries.
4. Any medical condition, take professional advice before
    practicing.

Akarna Dhanurasana(Chair Variation):

Akarna Dhanurasana, also known as the Archer's Bow Pose, is a
seated yoga pose that mimics the action of drawing a bow. This pose
stretches the shoulders, strengthens the legs, and improves spinal
mobility, helping to combat stiffness and enhance focus.

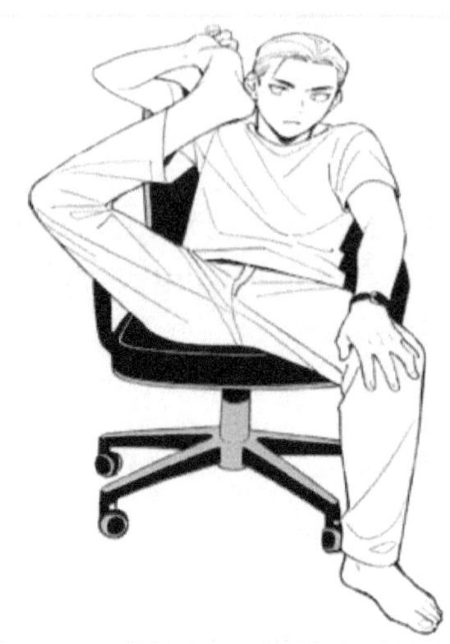

Steps:

1. Sit comfortably on a chair with your feet flat on the floor.
2. Keep your spine upright and shoulders relaxed.
3. Inhale and hold the right thumb finger and lift your right knee toward your chest, keeping your back straight.
4. Keep you left hand on left knee. If support needed for stability then you can hold right foot with your left hand.
5. Pull Like an Archer.
6. Pull your right foot slightly toward your right ear, mimicking the action of drawing an arrow.
7. Feel the stretch in your hip, hamstring, and shoulders.
8. Stay in this position for 15–30 seconds, breathing deeply.
9. Keep your gaze steady and your core engaged.
10. Exhale and slowly release the pose.
11. Repeat on the opposite side.

Benefits:

1. Counteracts the effects of prolonged sitting.
2. Stretches the arms and shoulders, reducing tension.
3. Engages muscles, improving circulation and mental clarity.

4. Activates the spine and abdominal muscles. Lower portion of the spine has been exercised.
5. Helps to move the bowels.

🚫 Contraindications:

Avoid if you have below health issues:
1. Severe knee or hip pain – Perform a milder stretch instead, based on your situation.
2. Lower back injuries – Avoid excessive pulling on the foot.
3. Recent shoulder injuries – Keep arm movements gentle.
4. Sciatica or herniated disc – Modify by reducing the leg lift.

Seated Virbhadrasana(Chair Variation):

Virabhadrasana (वीरभद्रासन) is named after Virabhadra, a fierce warrior created by Lord Shiva in Hindu mythology. Virabhadraasana also known as worrier pose. It's chair variation is very used full for the working peoples who does not get much time but want to take all most the similar benefits of traditional Virabhadrasana.

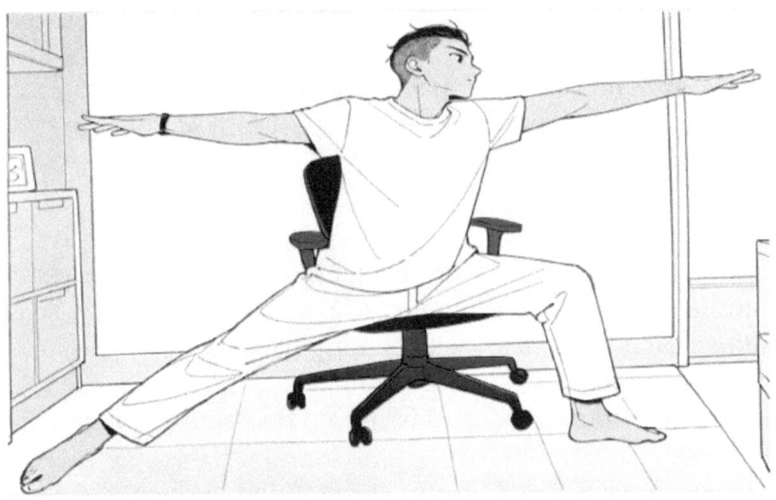

Steps:

1. Sit upright on a sturdy chair, feet flat on the ground, hip-width apart.
2. Keep your back straight and engage your core.

3. Shift to the right side of the chair, allowing your right thigh to face outward.
4. Extend your left leg sidewise, keeping your toes tucked under or resting on the top of your foot.
5. Keep your torso upright, engaging your abdominal muscles.
6. Square your hips forward as much as possible.
7. Inhale and raise and stretch your arms at shoulder level.
8. Keep your shoulders relaxed and chest open.
9. Stay in the pose for 15 to 30 seconds, feeling the stretch in your hips, chest, and shoulders.
10. Keep your gaze forward or slightly upward for a confident stance.

11. Exhale, bring your arms down, and return to a neutral seated position.
12. Repeat on the other side by shifting to the left edge of the chair and extending your right leg back.

Variations:

1. Raise your hand overhead, palms facing each other or joined.
2. Keep hands in Anjali Mudra (prayer position) at your chest.

Benefits:

1. Strengthens and stabilizes legs, hips, pelvis, spine, chest.
2. Relieves fatigue, back pain, asthma, arthritis, acidity, sciatica.
3. Practicing Virabhadrasana can improve mental focus and concentration
4. Enhances focus and mental clarity, boosting problem-solving skills.
5. Opens the chest and improves breathing, reducing stress and fatigue.

⊘ Contraindications:

1. Avoid if you have severe knee, hip, spinal or sholder injuries.
2. Do not overstretch, listen to your body and adjust accordingly.
3. Maintain even breathing and avoid tensing your shoulders.

Seated Marjaryasana Bitilasana(Seated Cat & Cow pose) – Chair variation:

Marjaryasana (Cat Pose) and Bitilasana (Cow Pose) are two complementary movements that gently stretch and mobilize the spine. In the chair variation, these poses are adapted for those who spend long hours sitting, making them ideal for software engineers and desk workers.

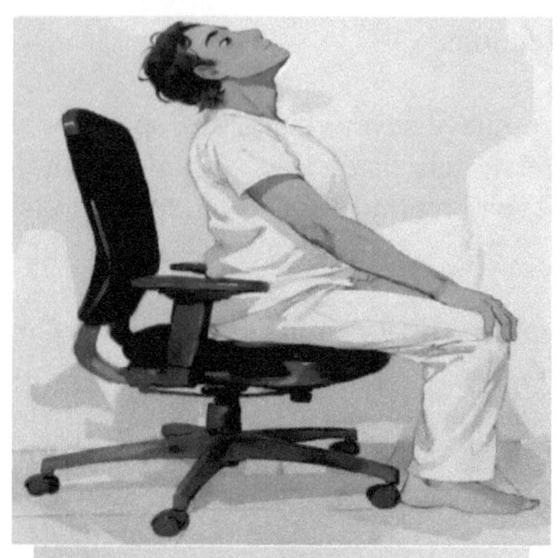

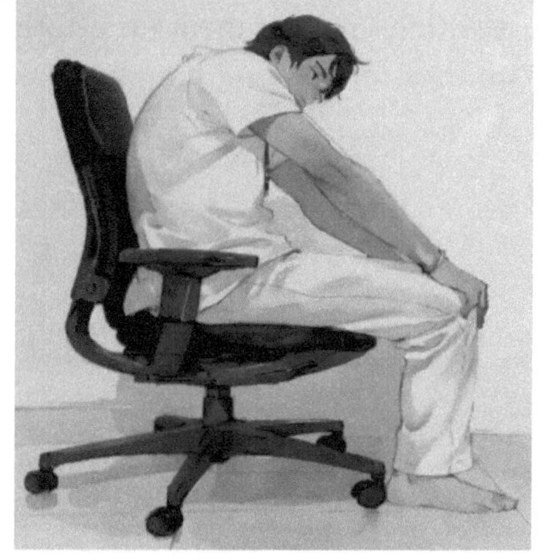

Steps:

1. Sit comfortably on a sturdy chair, feet flat on the ground, hip-width apart.
2. Keep your hands resting on your knees or thighs.
3. Maintain a straight spine with a neutral neck position.

Cow Pose (Bitilasana) – Inhale:

4. Arch your back, pushing your belly forward and lifting your chest.
5. Tilt your head slightly upward, opening the throat and stretching the neck.

6. Draw your shoulders back and down, engaging the upper back muscles.

Cat Pose (Marjaryasana) – Exhale:

7. Round your spine, tucking your chin toward your chest.
8. Pull your belly button inward, engaging the core muscles.
9. Press your hands against your knees for support, creating a deep stretch in the upper back.
10. Continue moving between Cow Pose (inhale, arching the back) and Cat Pose (exhale, rounding the spine) for 15 to 30 seconds, with mindful breaths.

Modifications & Variations:
11. For sensitive necks: Keep the head in a neutral position instead of tilting it back in Cow Pose.
12. For a deeper stretch: Add synchronized arm movements—lift the arms on the inhale and lower them on the exhale.

Benefits:

1. Relieves neck, shoulder, and lower back tension caused by long hours at the desk.
2. Improves spinal flexibility and posture alignment, reducing the risk of slouching.
3. Enhances breath awareness, helping reduce stress and improve focus.
4. Stimulates blood circulation, reduce hypertension, keeping the mind fresh and alert.

⊘ Contraindications:

1. Avoid if you have recent spinal injuries or severe back pain.
2. Move slowly and gently, keeping the movements smooth and controlled.
3. Breathe deeply, avoiding shallow or rushed breathing. High blood pressure.

Seated Navasana (Chair variation):

नवासन (Navasana) is a Sanskrit name. "Nava" means boat and "asana" means pose. So this pose makes the body resemble a boat floating on water, That's why it is called a Navasana.
Just like a well-balanced boat remains steady despite waves, a strong core helps us stay upright, balanced, and pain-free, even during long hours at a desk.

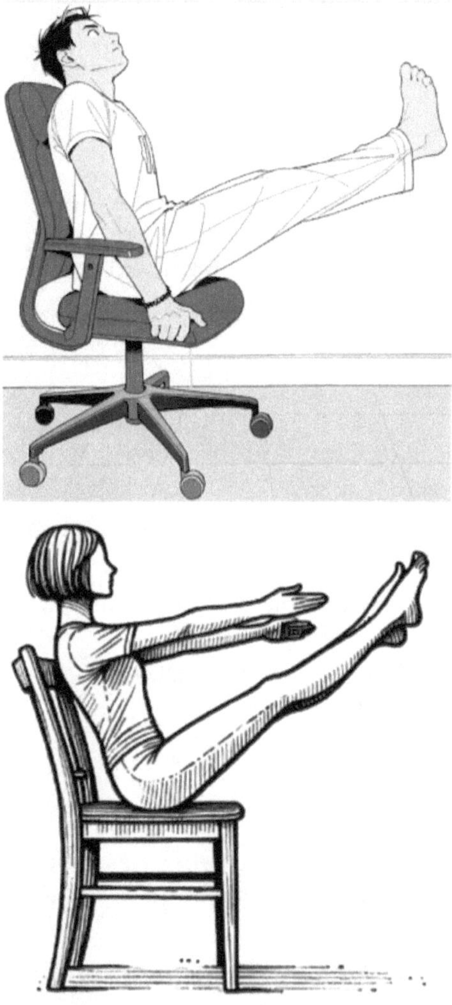

Steps:

Starting Position:

1. Sit at the edge of a sturdy chair with feet flat on the floor.
2. Keep your spine straight and engage your core muscles.

Lifting the Legs:

1. Lean back slightly while keeping your back straight.
2. Lift both feet off the ground, bringing the knees toward your chest.
3. Keep the legs bent at a 90-degree angle (for beginners) or extend them straight (for advanced practice).
4. If required you can hold the chair with your hand sidewise for better balance initially.

Engaging the Core:

1. Balance on your sitting bones, ensuring the core is actively engaged.
2. Extend your arms parallel to the floor, palms facing inward.
3. Keep your chest lifted and shoulders relaxed.

Holding the Pose:

1. Maintain this posture for 15-30 seconds, focusing on deep breathing.
2. Keep the abdominal muscles engaged throughout the hold.

Releasing the Pose:

1. Slowly lower your feet to the ground and sit upright.
2. Repeat 2/3 times if needed.

Benefits:

1. Strengthens the core muscles like abs, lower back, hip flexors.
2. Improves posture and spinal stability.
3. Boosts concentration and endurance.

1. Enhances digestion and metabolism, stimulates kidneys.
2. Reduces fat in abdominal area.

⊘ Contraindications:
1. Avoid if you have recent lower back injuries or abdominal surgery.
2. Do not strain the neck or shoulders, keep them relaxed.
3. Move slowly and engage the core, not the lower back.
4. Avoid when you have headache, heart problem and insomnia.

Seated Pavana Muktasana – Chair Variation:

This seated version of Pavana Muktasana is an excellent pose for digestion, spinal flexibility, and releasing lower back tension.

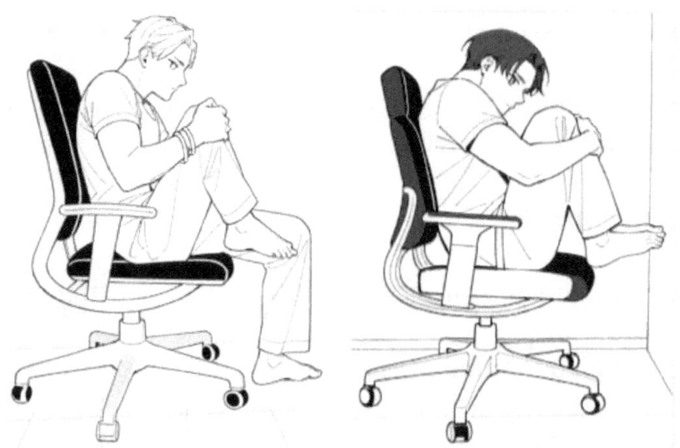

Steps to Perform:
1. Sit upright on chair, keeping both feet flat on the ground.
2. Lift your right knee towards your chest(Raise your right leg so that your knee moves toward your chest) and clasp your hands around your shin(Use both hands to hold the front part of your lower leg (the shin) just below the knee).
3. Gently pull the knee closer to your torso, keeping your spine tall.

4. Hold for 5-10 breaths, feeling a stretch in your lower back and hip.
5. Release slowly and switch to the left leg.
6. Now lift both knees together, hugging them toward your chest.

Benefits:
1. Releases lower back stiffness from prolonged sitting
2. Improves digestion (especially if working after meals)
3. Enhances blood circulation to prevent leg numbness
4. Easy to do at the desk without requiring much space

Contraindications:

Avoid if you have spine, knee injuries and abdominal issues.

Seated Ardha Matsyendrasana – Chair variation:

Ardha means half and Matsyendra means king of the fish. It known as 'Half Lord of the Fishes Pose'. Matsyendra" is one of the great Siddhas, who learned yoga from Lord Shiva while sitting inside a fish in deep meditation. Ardha Matsyendrasana is a classic spinal twist asana. Chair variation is very helpful for long sitting working guys.

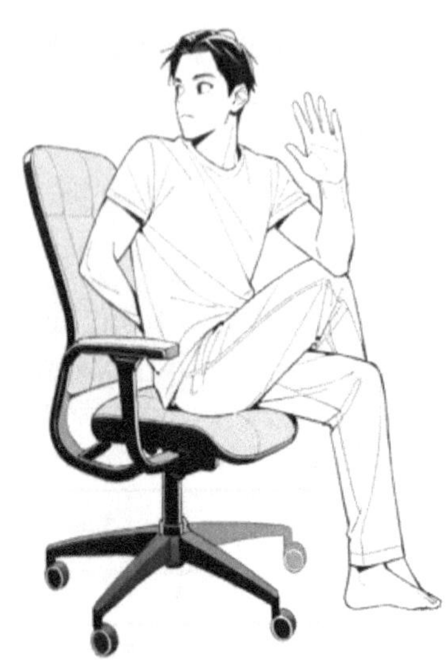

Steps:

1. Sit sideways on a chair with your feet flat on the ground.
2. Now you can cross your right leg on left thigh.
3. Place your right hand on the backrest of the chair or back of your body and your left hand on your right knee.
4. Inhale and lengthen your spine.
5. Exhale and gently twist your torso to the right, looking over your shoulder.
6. Hold in this pose for 15/20 seconds, feeling the stretch along your spine.
7. Return to the center and repeat on the other side.

Benefits:
1. Relieves stiffness from prolonged sitting.
2. Improves spinal mobility and posture.
3. Enhances digestion and circulation.
4. Reduces stress and mental fatigue.
5. Get relief from lower back pain.
6. Improve sleep pattern.

🚫 Contraindications:

Avoid if you have severe back pain and injuries. Abdominal
injuries.

Seated Padahastasana (Chair variation):

Padahastasana is standing forward bending posture. Pada means
foot and hasta means hand.
Seated Padahastasana, or the Seated Hand-to-Foot Pose, is a simple
yet effective yoga posture.

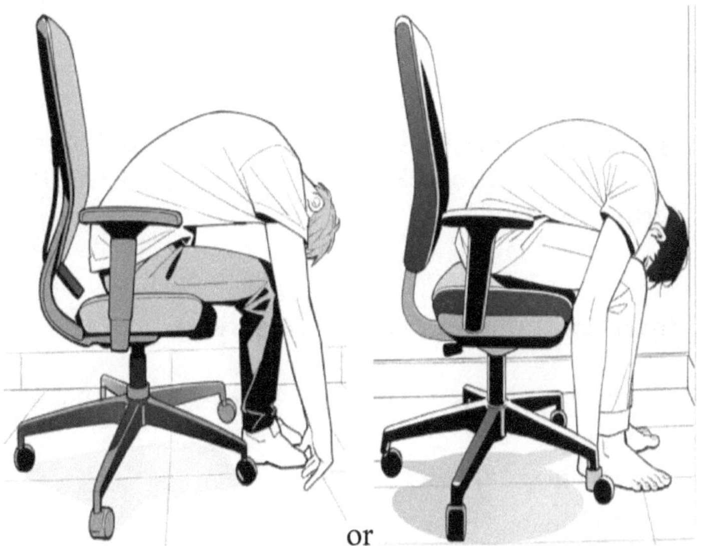

Steps:

1. Sit on a chair with feet flat on the floor, hip-width apart.
2. Inhale deeply and lengthen your spine, keeping your back
   straight.
3. As you are inhaling rise your hand straight above your head.
4. Exhale and slowly bend forward from your hips, reaching your
   hands toward your feet or the floor.
5. Let your head and neck relax, allowing gravity to deepen the
   stretch.
6. Hold this position for 15/20 seconds, with normal breathing.
7. To release, inhale and slowly return to an upright position.

Benefits:

1. Great asana for hamstring and wrist stretch.
2. Relieves back tension from prolonged sitting.
3. Helps preventing constipation and menstrual problems.
4. Improves flexibility in the hamstrings and lower back.
5. Boosts blood circulation to the brain, enhancing focus and reducing mental fatigue.
6. Encourages mindfulness, helping to reduce stress and improve posture awareness.
7. improves the blood flow to the pancreas. Improves digestion.

🚫 Contraindications:

Avoid if you have severe back pain and injuries. Abdominal injuries. High or Low Blood Pressure. Glaucoma or Eye Pressure Issues. Vertigo or Dizziness

Seated Paschimottanasana (Chair variation):

"Paschima" (पश्चिम) Means "West" or "Backside" (referring to the back of the body).
"Uttana" (उत्तान) Means "Intense Stretch."
"Asana" (आसन) Means "Pose."
Thus it is why Paschimottanasana translate as "Intense Stretch of the Backside of the Body".

In the traditional Paschimottanasana, you sit with your legs stretched straight in front and fold forward from the hips, trying to reach your feet. The Chair modification replicates the same movement but is adapted for those who cannot sit on the floor and accessible to those who work at desks, offering spinal relief without needing to leave their seats.

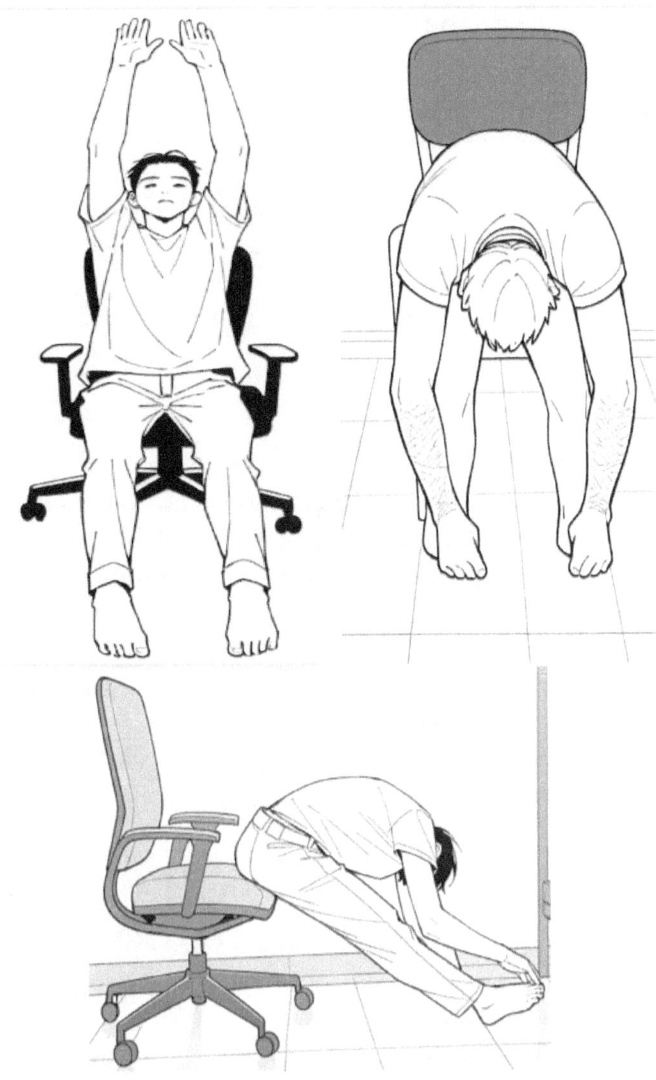

Steps:

1. Sit comfortably on a chair with your feet stretched forward on the floor, hip-width apart. Keep your spine straight and shoulders relaxed.
2. Inhale deeply, lengthening your spine, reaching your arms overhead.

3. Exhale and begin to fold forward from your hips, reaching your hands towards your feet or ankles. If flexibility allows, hold the sides of your feet.
4. Allow your head to relax towards your knees, keeping the neck long and tension-free.
5. Breathe normally and hold the stretch for 20-30 seconds, feeling the release along your spine, lower back, and hamstrings.
6. Inhale slowly and come back up to a seated position with a straight spine.

Benefits:

1. Releases lower back tension caused by prolonged sitting.
2. Improves spinal flexibility and prevents stiffness.
3. Enhances digestion by stimulating abdominal organs.
4. Reduces stress and calms the mind, nerves system and improving focus.
5. Increases circulation to the pelvic region. It stimulates the circulation into the nerves.
6. Massages and tones the abdominal and pelvic organs and stimulates insulin production. So good for diabetes.

⃠ Contraindications:

1. Don't try beyond your body limits.
2. Avoid if you have severe back injuries or slipped disc issues. Abdominal injuries.
3. Those with high blood pressure or vertigo should perform it with caution, keeping the head elevated.

Seated Gomukhasana - Chair Variation:

Gomukhasana, or Cow Face Pose, is a yoga posture that deeply stretches the shoulders, chest, arms, hips, and thighs. The name came from Sanskrit:
"Go" = Cow
"Mukha" = Face

"Asana" = Pose

When performed, the crossed legs resemble a cow's face, and the arms mimic its ears.

Chair Variation is an effective stretch to open the shoulders, improve posture, and relieve tension in the upper body without leaving your working desk.

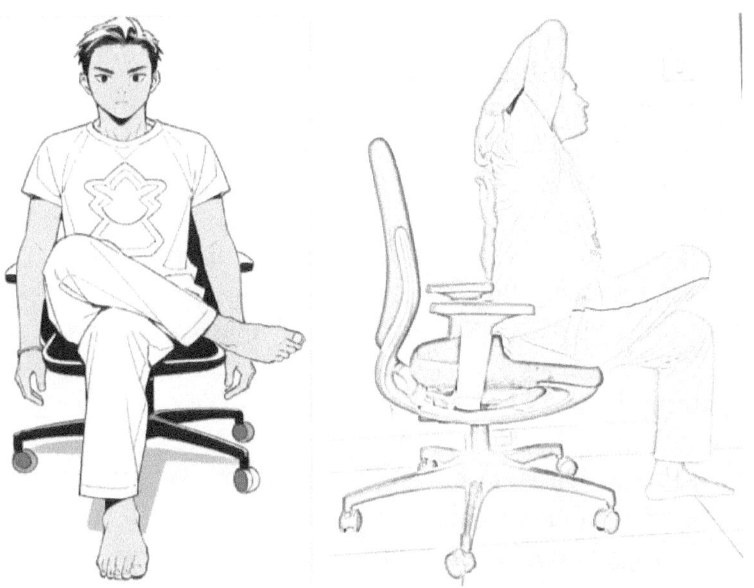

Steps:

1. Sit comfortably on a chair with your feet flat on the ground and spine straight.
2. Now Cross your right leg over your left, if possible place the right foot near your left hip.
3. Raise your right arm overhead and bend the elbow, allowing the hand to reach down behind your upper back.
4. Bring your left arm behind your back and try to clasp your right fingers.
5. If your hands don't reach each other, use a towel, or handkerchief to bridge the gap.
6. Keep your chest open, shoulders relaxed, and spine tall.
7. Maintain this posture for 20/30 seconds while breathing normally.

8. Feel the stretch in the shoulders, triceps, and upper back.
9. Release the hands, Switch Sides and repeat the same steps with the opposite arm on top.

Benefits:

1. Relieves Shoulder & Neck Tension – Reduces stiffness from prolonged typing and mouse usage.
2. Improves Posture – Counteracts slouching and rounded shoulders caused by screen time.
3. Enhances Flexibility – Opens the chest and stretches the spine, keeping the upper body agile.
4. Boosts Circulation – Encourages better blood flow to the arms and shoulders, preventing fatigue.
5. Improves back pain, anxiety and neuro problems.

🚫 Contraindications:

1. Shoulder or Rotator Cuff Injuries – Avoid if you have severe shoulder pain.
2. Frozen Shoulder or Arthritis – Modify the stretch by using a strap.
3. Lower Back Strain – Ensure the spine remains upright to avoid pressure on the lower back.

Seated Marichyasana- Chair variation:

Marichyasana is named after the sage Marichi, meaning "ray of light" in Sanskrit. It involves a deep spinal twist or forward bend, depending on the variation. The Chair Variation of Marichyasana is an adapted version that makes the pose accessible to individuals who spend long hours sitting, such as software engineers.

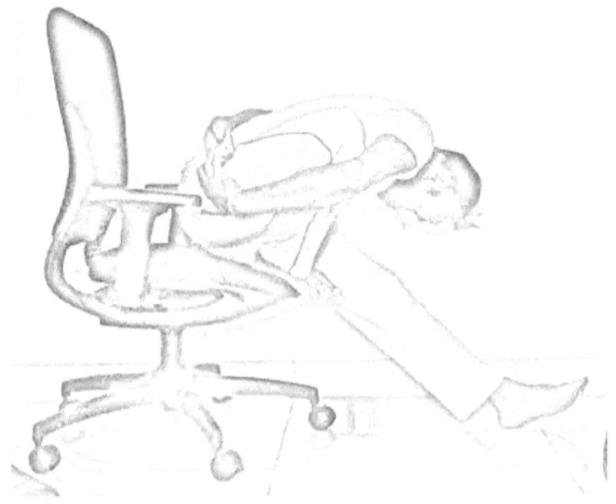

Steps:

1. Sit upright on a chair with your feet flat on the ground and knees hip-width apart.
2. Keep your spine elongated and shoulders relaxed.
3. Now slightly straight your left leg forward.
4. Bend your right knee and place the right foot firmly on the seat of the chair.
5. Bring your left hand behind you and right hand through rounding your right leg towards back and try to hold both hand.
6. Inhale and bend forward.
7. Hold this posture for 20-30 seconds, then slowly come back.
8. Repeat on the other side.

Option 2:
Other than bending forward here you can twist right side backward.

Benefits:
1. Enhances spinal flexibility and mobility.
2. Relieves stiffness in the lower back, shoulders, and neck.
3. Aids digestion and stimulates internal organs.
4. Improves posture and helps counteract the effects of prolonged sitting.
5. Promotes relaxation and reduces stress.

1. Avoid if you have spinal disc injuries or severe lower back pain.
2. Be cautious if you have recent abdominal surgery or digestive issues.
3. If you experience discomfort in the knees or hips, use a cushion for support.

Ardha Chakrasana chair variation:

Sanskrit words Ardha meaning Half and Chakra meaning wheel, so Ardha Chakrasana means half wheel deep back bending. In the chair variation, this asana is adapted for seated practitioners, making it more accessible for office workers, seniors, or those with mobility challenges.

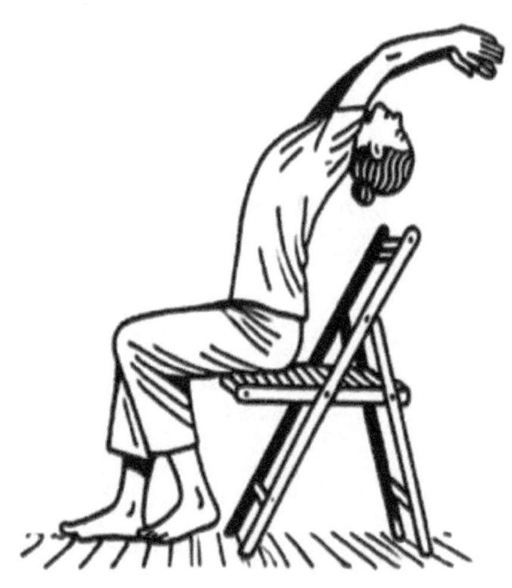

Steps:

1. Sit comfortably on a sturdy chair with your feet flat on the floor, hip-width apart.

2. Keep your spine straight and hands resting on your thighs.
3. Place your hands on your lower back or the sides of the chair for support.
4. Inhale deeply bend your body backward and gently lift your chest upward.
5. Slowly arch your upper back, allowing your head to tilt slightly backward.
6. Keep your elbows drawn inward, engaging your back muscles.
7. Focus on lengthening the spine rather than just bending.
8. Maintain the pose for 20/30 seconds, breaths normally without straining.
9. Keep your core engaged and avoid compressing the lower back.
10. Exhale and slowly return to an upright seated position.
11. Rest for a few breaths before repeating if needed.

Option 2 (Alternative Hand Position):

You can also place your hand as below position: at point 3 hand position can be changed as
Breathing in, extend your arms overhead with your palms facing each other.

Benefits:

1. Improves spinal flexibility and posture.
2. Opens the chest and shoulders, enhancing lung capacity.
3. Relieves mild back pain and stiffness.
4. Helps counteract the effects of prolonged sitting.
5. Stimulates energy and alertness, reducing fatigue.
6. Opens the chest, strengthens the spine, and improves flexibility.

🚫 Contraindications:

1. People with severe lower back pain or recent spinal injuries.

2. Those with dizziness, vertigo, or high blood pressure should perform with caution.
3. Avoid if experiencing abdominal discomfort.
4. Avoid if you have High blood pressure. Hernia.

Half Frog chair pose:

The Half Frog Chair Pose is a gentle seated variation of the traditional Ardha Bhekasana (Half Frog Pose). It is designed for individuals who spend long hours at a desk, helping to open the hip flexors, stretch the quadriceps, and improve spinal mobility while being seated. This makes it an ideal yoga posture for software engineers and desk workers.

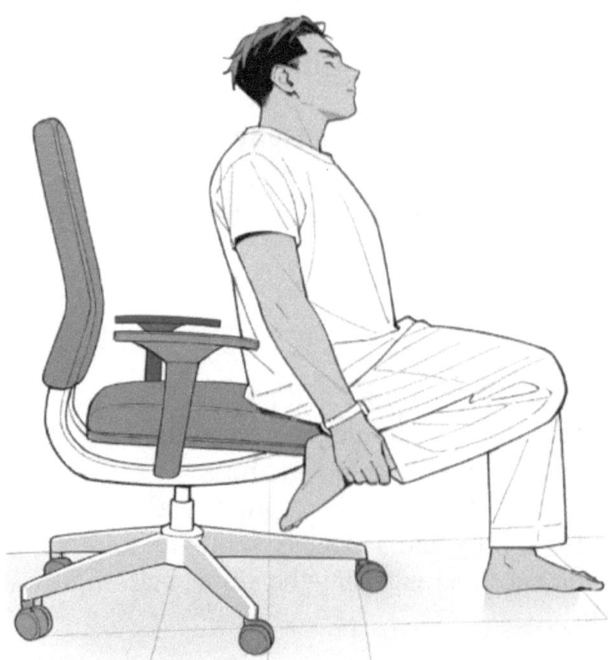

Steps:

1. Sit upright on a chair with both feet flat on the ground.
2. Shift your weight slightly to one side and bring your right knee back, allowing your right foot to move behind you.

3. Hold your right ankle with your right hand, gently pulling it towards your glute.
4. Keep your chest open and your left foot planted firmly on the ground.
5. Engage your core and ensure that your lower back is not overarched.
6. Hold the position for 15-20 seconds, breathing deeply.
7. Release the leg slowly and return to the seated position.
8. Repeat on the other side.

Benefits:

1. Stretches the quadriceps, hip flexors, and psoas muscles.
2. Relieves tension from prolonged sitting.
3. Enhances spinal flexibility.
4. Improves posture and counteracts the effects of slouching.
5. Helps with knee and ankle mobility.

⊘ Contraindications:
1. Avoid if you have knee or lower back injuries.
2. If you experience discomfort, use a strap or modify the pose to avoid strain.

Seated Prone Stretch (Sphinx Pose - Chair Variation):

The Seated Prone Stretch, inspired by the Sphinx Pose in yoga, is a gentle backbend performed on a chair. It helps in stretching the spine, opening the chest, and relieving tension in the back and shoulders. This pose also is particularly beneficial for software engineers who spend long hours sitting, as it counteracts the effects of poor posture and prolonged screen time.

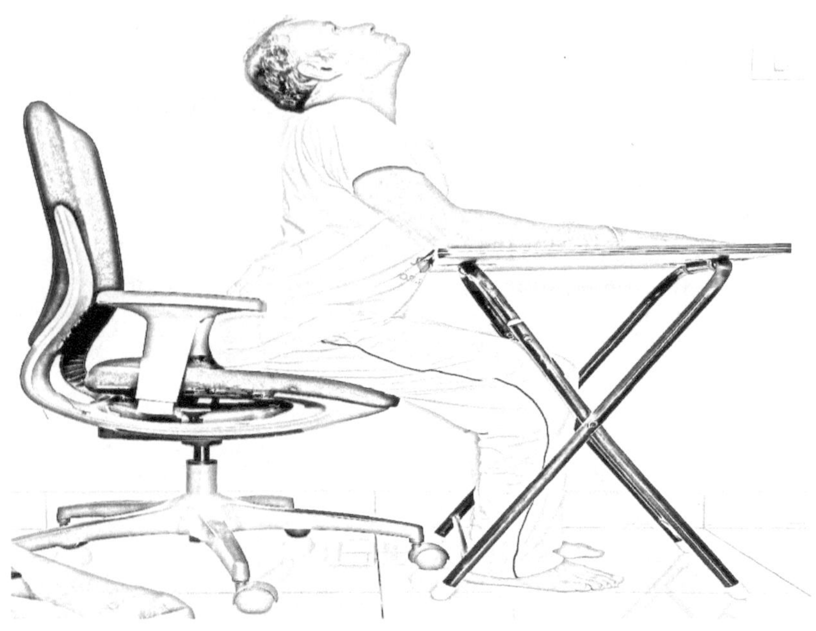

Steps:

1. Sit comfortably on a sturdy chair with your feet flat on the ground and hip-width apart. Keep your back straight and hands resting on your thighs.
2. Place your forearms on the desk in front of you, keeping your elbows aligned under your shoulders. Your palms should be facing down, creating a 90-degree angle with your arms.
3. Inhale and lift your chest slightly, allowing a gentle curve in your lower back. Keep your head in line with your spine and avoid straining your neck.
4. Hold this position for 15/20 deep breaths, allowing your chest to open and your back muscles to engage.
5. Exhale and gently relax your body, bringing your arms back to your lap.

Benefits:

1. Relieves tension in the lower back and spine.
2. Opens the chest and shoulders, improving posture.
3. Enhances blood circulation to the upper body.

4. Reduces stress and fatigue from prolonged desk work.

⊘ Contraindications:

1. Avoid this pose if you have severe lower back pain or spinal injuries.
2. Do not overstretch; keep movements gentle and controlled.
3. Maintain proper chair support to avoid excessive strain on the lower back.

Bakasana/Crow Pose on a Chair:

Seated Crow Pose on a Chair, is a modified version of the traditional Bakasana (Crow Pose) that provides the benefits of arm balance while being accessible for individuals who may have difficulty performing the full version on the floor. This variation is ideal for office workers, software engineers, or anyone who spends long hours sitting, as it strengthens the arms, core, and wrists while improving focus and balance.

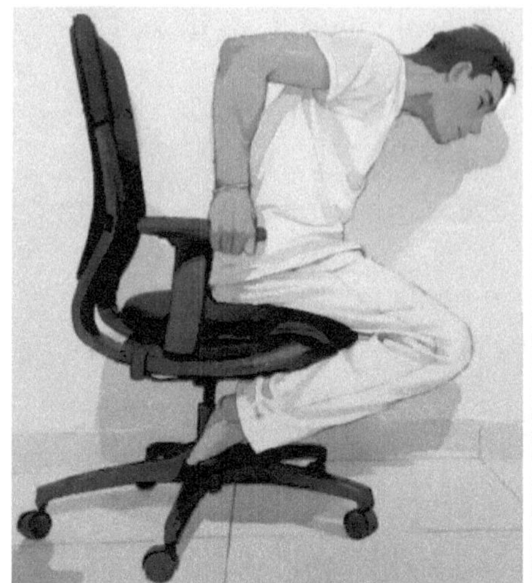 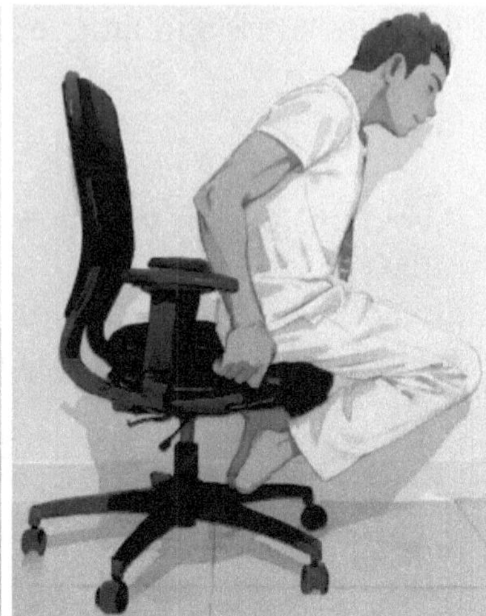

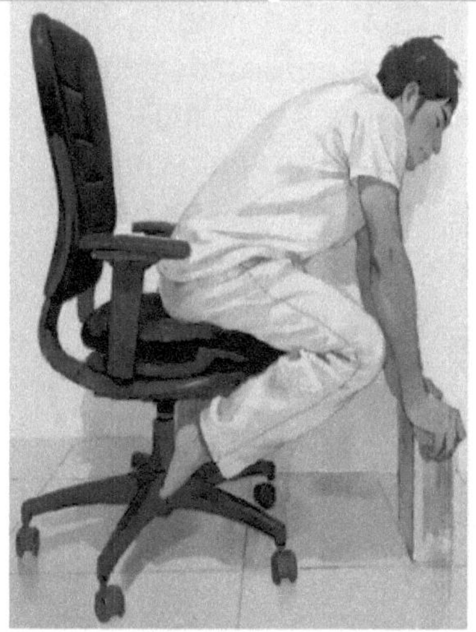

Steps:

1. Sit on the edge of a sturdy chair with your feet flat on the floor, hip-width apart.
2. Place your hands on the seat of the chair, shoulder-width apart, fingers pointing forward, and spread your fingers for a strong grip.
3. Engage your core and lift onto your toes, bringing your knees close to your upper arms or triceps.
4. Lean slightly forward, shifting your body weight onto your hands while keeping your elbows bent.

5. Lift one foot off the floor, then the other, finding balance as you engage your abdominal muscles. Don't touch the chair by toe.
6. Squeeze your knees toward your upper arms and hold the position for a few breaths, keeping your gaze forward.
7. To release, gently bring your feet back to the floor and sit back on the chair.

Option:
You can put some height down on the flow and bend and put your palm on it as 3rd pic

Benefits:

1. Strengthens the arms, wrists, and core for better posture and endurance.
2. Enhances focus and concentration, improving mental clarity.
3. Promotes wrist flexibility, reducing the risk of repetitive strain injuries from typing.
4. Encourages balance and coordination, improving body awareness.

Contraindications:

Avoid if you have wrist, elbow, or shoulder injuries.
Do not practice if you have high blood pressure or severe lower back pain.
Always use a stable chair without wheels for safety.
Pregnant individuals or those with recent surgeries should consult a doctor before attempting.

Seated Cobra Pose (Bhujangasana - Chair Variation for Back Relief):

Bhujangasana, also known as Cobra Pose, is a reclining backbend in yoga that resembles a cobra raising its hood. It's a prone asana. It is performed by lying on the stomach and lifting the upper body using the support of the hands while keeping the legs and lower body grounded. This pose helps in strengthening the spine, opening the chest, and improving flexibility.

In a chair variation, the same principles apply, but the person sits on a chair and leans back, using the hands for support while arching the spine and lifting the chest.

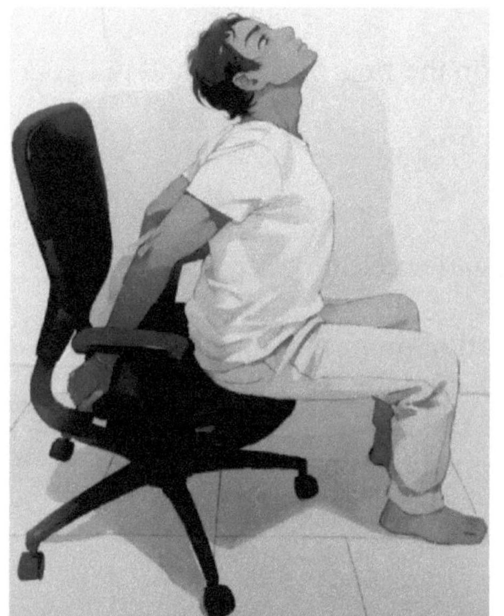 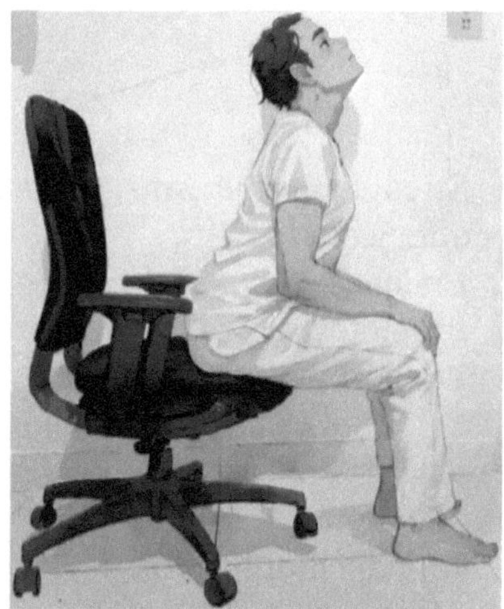

Steps:

1. Sit on a sturdy chair with your back straight and feet flat on the floor, hip-width apart.
2. Place your hands on the back edge of the chair seat, fingers pointing downward. Ensure your arms are slightly behind your hips.
3. As you inhale, press your hands into the chair and arch your back gently. Lift your chest upward and roll your shoulders back.
4. Head and Neck Position: Allow your head to tilt slightly backward, looking upward if comfortable, keeping your neck relaxed.

5. Maintain this position for 20-30 seconds with normal/deep breathing, feeling a stretch in your chest, shoulders, and upper abdomen.
6. Exhale and slowly return to a neutral sitting position. Repeat if needed.

Benefits:

1. Stretches the chest, shoulders, and abdomen.
2. Strengthens the lower back and improves spinal flexibility.
3. Helps counteract slouching and promotes better posture.
4. Enhances lung capacity and deepens breathing.
5. Reduces the stress, hypertension.

Contraindications:

1. Avoid excessive back bending if you have lower back pain.
2. Avoid if you have abdominal issues or any recent surgery.
3. Avoid if you have heart disease or high blood pressure.

Seated Reverse Prayer Pose (Paschima Namaskarasana - Chair Variation):

Paschima Namaskarasana (Reverse Prayer Pose) - Chair Variation is a seated yoga posture that involves bringing the hands behind the back in a reverse prayer position. This pose enhances flexibility in the shoulders, chest, and wrists while promoting better posture and mindfulness. The chair variation makes the pose accessible for individuals with mobility restrictions, allowing them to experience the benefits of the asana while maintaining spinal alignment and comfort.

Paschima means west but here it's backside.
Namskara means greeting and
Asana means pose.

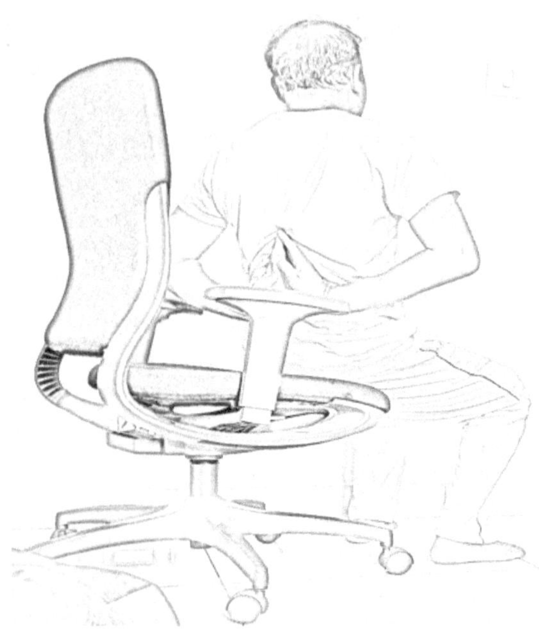

Steps:

1. Sit comfortably on a chair with your feet firmly planted on the ground, hip-width apart.
2. Keep your spine tall and shoulders relaxed.
3. Bring your hands behind your back and press your palms together in a reverse prayer position (Paschima Namaskara).
4. If this is challenging, you can hold opposite elbows or rest your hands on your lower back.
5. Roll your shoulders back and gently press your palms together to open the chest.
6. Keep your wrists aligned and fingers pointing upward.
7. Maintain a slight engagement in the core for support.
8. Inhale deeply, expanding the chest while maintaining a straight spine.
9. Exhale slowly, allowing the shoulders to relax without collapsing the chest.
10. Stay in this position for 20/30 seconds with deep/normal breathing, focusing on the stretch across the chest and shoulders.

11. If comfortable, slightly tilt your chin upward for a deeper chest opening.
12. Exhale as you gently separate your hands and bring them forward.
13. Shake out your arms to release any tension.

Benefits:

1. Enhances flexibility and mobility in the shoulders and wrists.
2. Improves posture and reduces tension in the upper back.
3. Encourages deep breathing and relaxation.
4. Aids in stress relief and mental clarity.

🚫 Contraindications:

Avoid if you have low blood pressure, arm or shoulder injury.

Seated Kurmasana (Tortoise Pose - Chair Variation):

Kurmasana (Tortoise Pose) is a deep forward fold that stretches the spine, shoulders, and hamstrings while calming the mind. In a chair variation, it can be modified to provide almost the similar benefits while being accessible for office workers and software engineers.

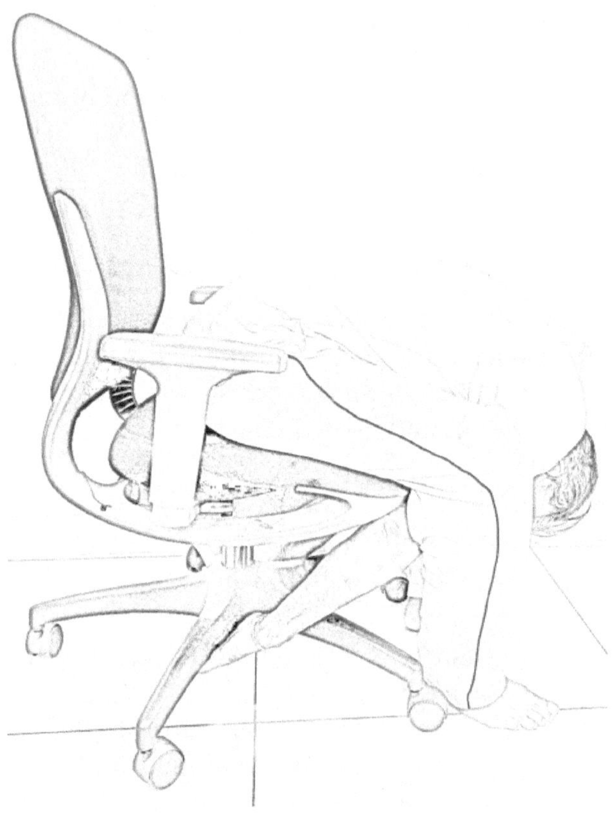

Steps to Perform Seated Kurmasana on a Chair

1. Sit at the Edge of the Chair
   - Keep feet flat on the floor, hip-width apart.
   - Sit upright with a straight spine.
2. Widen the Legs
   - Spread your legs slightly wider than hip-width, keeping knees bent at 90 degrees.
   - Allow enough space for your torso to fold forward.
3. Hinge at the Hips & Fold Forward
   - Inhale, lengthen the spine.
   - Exhale, slowly hinge forward from the hips, bringing the torso down between the thighs.
4. Slide Arms Under Legs
   - Extend arms forward, then slide them under the thighs, reaching toward the back.

o   Keep palms facing downward or clasp hands behind your back for a deeper stretch.

5. **Relax the Neck & Breathe**
    o   Let the head drop naturally, keeping the neck relaxed.
    o   Hold for 5-10 deep breaths, feeling the stretch along the spine and shoulders.

6. **Release Gently**
    o   Inhale, engage your core, and slowly lift your torso back up.
    o   Bring legs together and rest hands on the thighs.

Benefits of Seated Kurmasana on a Chair for Software Engineers

o   Relieves tension in the spine from prolonged sitting.
o   Stretches the shoulders and wrists, reducing strain from typing.
o   Calms the nervous system, helping with mental clarity.
o   Opens the hips, counteracting stiffness from sitting all day
o   As per B.K.S. Iyengar in Light on Yoga, "tones the spine, activates the abdominal organs, and keeps one energetic and healthy."

🚫 Contraindications:

Avoid if you have severe back pain and injuries. Abdominal injuries. High or Low Blood Pressure. Vertigo or Dizziness.

Seated Ustrasana (Camel Pose) on a Chair:

The Ustrasana (Camel Pose) Chair Variant is a great heart-opening and backbend posture adapted for seated practice.

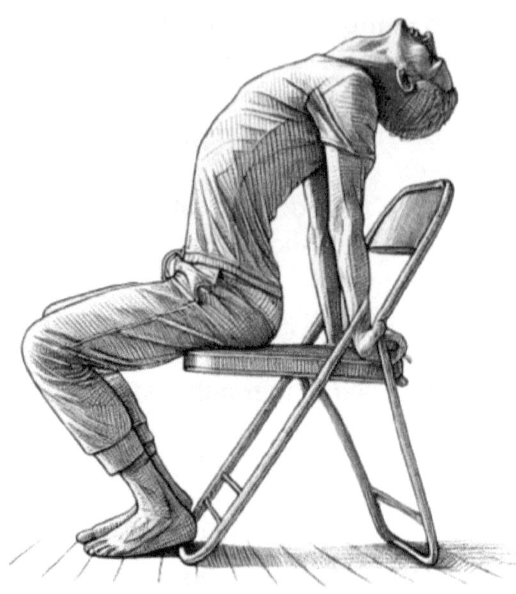

1. Sit at the edge of the chair with feet flat on the ground and hip-width apart.
2. Place your hands on the chair's backrest or the sides of the seat for support.
3. Inhale, lift your chest, and arch your spine backward, keeping your core engaged.
4. Option 1: Keep hands on the chair's backrest for gentle support.
5. Option 2: Reach your arms back, holding the chair legs for a deeper stretch.
6. Gently drop your head back, only if comfortable, to enhance the heart-opening effect.
7. Hold for 3-5 breaths, then slowly return to an upright position.

Benefits:
   o   Stretches the chest, shoulders, and front body
   o   Strengthens the back and improves posture
   o   Enhances lung capacity and relieves tension

🚫 Contraindications:

Avoid if you have severe back pain and injuries and shoulder injuries. Abdominal injuries. Vertigo or Dizziness.

Setu Bandhasana (Bridge Pose) – Chair Variation:

Setu Bandhasana called as Bridge pose as it'll create a bridge like arche. A formation of bridge. This seated variation of Setu Bandhasana (Bridge Pose) is excellent for opening the chest, strengthening the back, and improving posture, making it ideal for software engineers who spend long hours sitting.

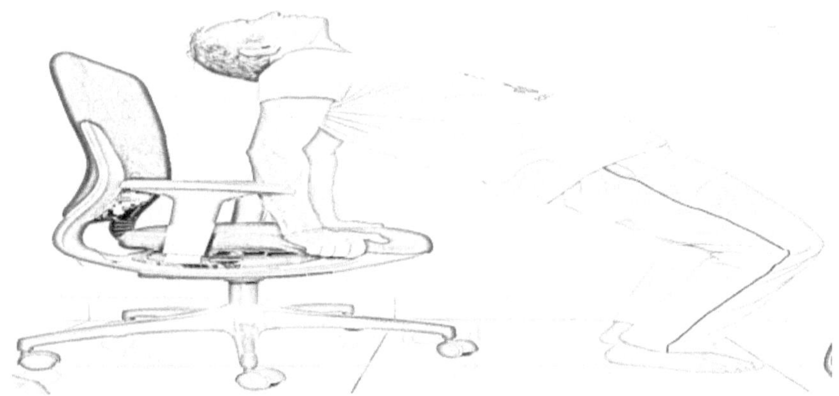

Steps to Perform:
1. Sit at the edge of the chair, keeping your feet flat on the floor and hip-width apart.
2. Hold the sides of the chair seat for stability.
3. Press your feet firmly into the ground and engage your glutes.
4. Lift your hips upward, arching your back slightly.
5. Open your chest and slightly tilt your head back while keeping your neck relaxed.
6. Maintain the posture for 10 -15 seconds, then slowly lower your hips back down.

Benefits:
1. Strengthens the back & glutes, reducing lower back pain.
2. Improves posture & circulation, preventing stiffness.

3. Relieves depression and anxiety.
4. The lungs are opened up, and thyroid problems are reduced.
5. The lungs are opened up, and thyroid problems are reduced.

◎ Contraindications:
Avoid practicing when you have below issues:
1. Neck or Spine Injuries.
2. Recent Surgery.
3. Severe Knee Pain.
4. High Blood Pressure. Or Any other medical issue.

Chapter 4

Pranayama chair variations

Pranayama

Patanjali describes Pranayama is regulation of breath, breath control. When we inhale we take vital energy inside and with the exhale we remove the waste and toxins out from physical body and mind. Puraka is a state of Pranayama where in one gets air through nostril which is held inside the lungs with a pause. Kumbhaka is an interval or suspension of breath for some time between inhalation and exhalation. The retention of breathing after inhale is called Abhyanta Kumbhaka and retention of breath after exhalation is called Bhahya Kumbhaka. Recaka is a state of Pranayama where in one expels the air from inside one's lungs. Pranayama is the heart of yoga. The word prana is composed of two words, pra and na. Pra means 'first unit' and na means 'energy'. Prana is the sum total of all energy that is manifest in man and the universe. It was said by the ancient sages, "one who knows the science of breath knows everything and he knows prana knows the vedas".

Why to Integrate Pranayama into Your Workday:
1. Morning Energizer:
    o Practice Kapalabhati or Bhastrika for a quick energy boost.
2. Midday Stress Relief:
    o Use Nadi Shodhana or Bhramari or Chandra nadi to calm your mind and reset your focus.
3. Post-Work Relaxation:
    o Ujjayi or Sitali helps cool down your mind and body after a long day.
4. Short Breaks:
    o Incorporate Nadi Shodhana or Shuni Mudra with Pranayama for 3-5 minutes to stay balanced during breaks.

Initially started with Natural Breath Awareness:

Natural Breath Awareness is a simple technique which anyone can do. It's a wonderful way to begin your own pranayama practice, checking in with how your feeling at any given moment in time and then feel the benefits of breathing practices for yourself. Start by sitting or lying in any comfortable position, and take some time to settle in. Then:

- Begin to notice the breath. How does it feel? Is it shallow, or deep; fast, or slow? Is there any tension in the breath?
- Keep noticing. Become aware of the temperature of the breath: coolness on the inhalation, and warmth on the exhalation.
- Follow the pathway of the breath from nose all the way to the abdomen.
- As you become increasingly aware of the rhythm of your breath, don't try to change it.

Preparatory Breathing Practice:

Sit on chair comfortably, Spine will be straight and erected.

The head, neck, and back should be aligned. Abdominal muscles and shoulder muscles should be relaxed.

Place your hand on thighs or knees with chin mudra.

Now close your eyes and take deep a inhale through nose and deep exhale through nose. Exhale should be more than inhale(approximately inhale : exhale as 1:2). Be aware for your breathing.

Practice this for around 5 minutes.

Yogic Breathing(Sectional Breathing):

Yogic Breathing, also known as Sectional Breathing or Dirgha Pranayama, involves consciously expanding different sections of the lungs-the abdomen, rib cage, and upper chest-in a sequential manner. This type of breathing helps to utilize the lungs fully, promoting deep relaxation and revitalizing energy. For IT professionals, who often face mental fatigue, mental hygiene issues, poor posture, and shallow breathing due to prolonged desk work, Yogic Breathing offers a simple and effective way to improve well-being. Rapid breathing, shallow breathing create s negative impact on our body, and mind which can translate to nervousness, stress, pain and tensions. So all exercises in yoga and breathing exercises, pranayama should be performed gently with full awareness. So yogic breathing can restore our breathing patterns and improves a healthy breathing practice.

The full yogic breathing involves the three types of breathing; abdominal breathing, chest/thoracic breathing, and collarbone breathing.

Practice:
1. Sit comfortably on chair with Spine will be straight and erected. Feet flat on the floor, and hands resting on your knees or lap.
2. During Practice you can close your eyes also.

3. Abdominal Breathing:

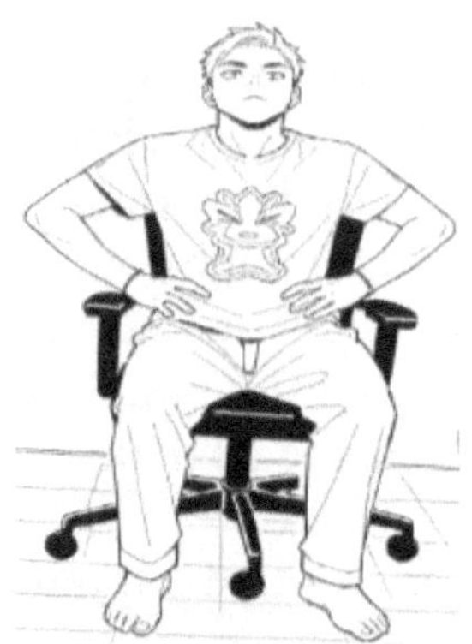

- o Place your hand on your belly with fingers pointed toward navel, mainly middle finger towards navel and other finger can be stretch out either side, but should not press the belly.
- o Inhale slowly through the nose, expanding the abdomen outward.
- o Exhale fully, allowing the abdomen to contract.
- o Focus on the rise and fall of the belly.
- o Repeat for 5-10 breaths.

4. Thoracic (Rib Cage) Breathing:

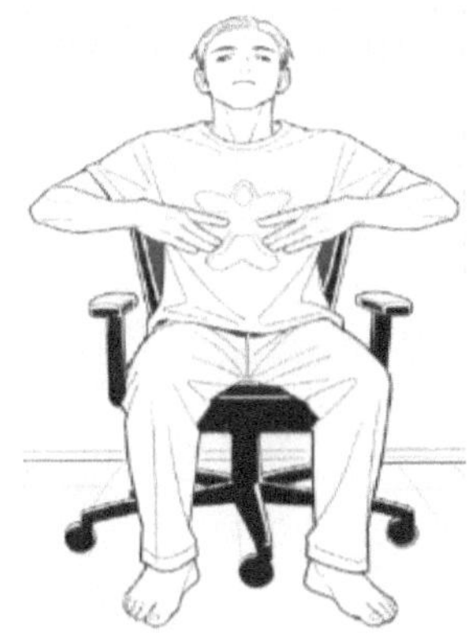

- o Place your hands lightly on your rib cage with fingers stretched out. Little finger should be placed on lower rib case. The thumb finger should face armpits at the top of the rib case.
- o Inhale slowly, expanding the rib cage outward and upward.
- o Exhale, allowing the ribs to return to their original position.
- o Avoid moving the abdomen.
- o Repeat for 5-10 breaths.

5. Clavicular (Collarbone) Breathing:

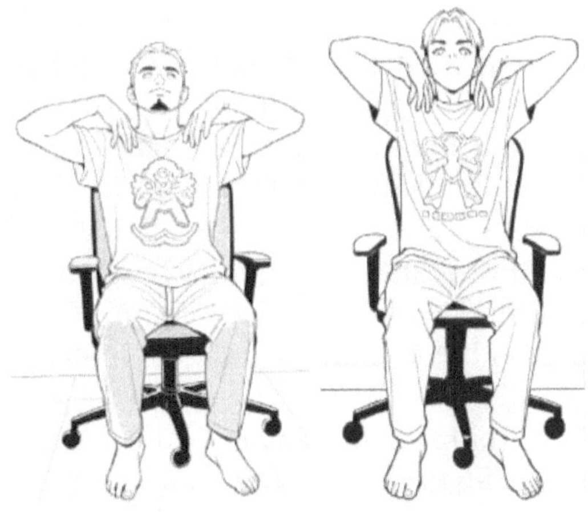

- o Place your fingertips gently on your collarbones.

- o Inhale deeply, lifting the collarbones and expanding the upper chest.
- o Exhale, allowing the upper chest to relax.
- o Repeat for 5-10 breaths.

6. Full Yogic Breath:

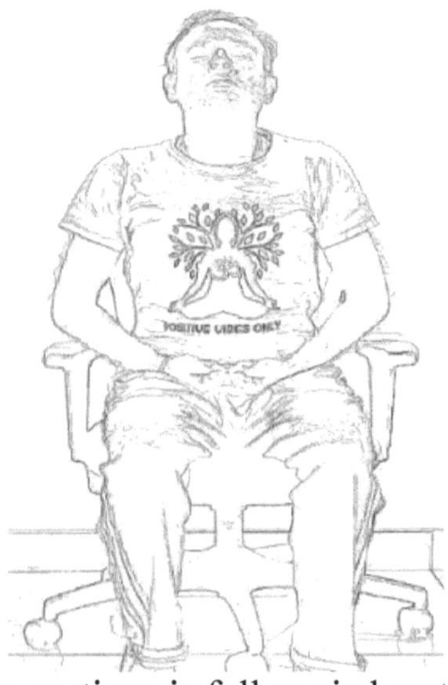

- o Combine all three sections is full yogic breath.
- o Place your hand on your knees or lap with brahma mudra or simply pump facing downward or upwards.
- o Inhale first into the abdomen, then expand the rib cage, and finally lift the upper chest and collarbones.
- o Retain your breath for few seconds.
- o Start exhaling slowly in reverse order, by relaxing the upper chest, then the rib cage, and finally the abdomen.
- o Ensure the breath is smooth and continuous.
- o Repeat for 5-10 full breaths.

Finally relax and breath normally for a minutes.

Benefits for working Professionals:
- o Reduces Stress and Anxiety
- o Promotes deep relaxation, calming the nervous system.
- o Improves Focus, thinking power and Clarity.

- o Enhances oxygen supply to the brain, reducing mental fatigue.
- o Corrects Poor Posture
- o Encourages full lung expansion, which counteracts the effects of slouched sitting.
- o Combats Sedentary Fatigue
- o Refreshes the mind and body by increasing oxygenation.
- o Helps release tightness in the shoulders and chest.
- o Improves Breathing Efficiency
- o Strengthens lung capacity and encourages full, mindful breathing.

Seated Dog Breathing (Chair Variation):

This chair yoga pose helps relieve tension in the shoulders, spine, and lower back while promoting deep breathing. It is ideal for software engineers who spend long hours sitting at a desk.

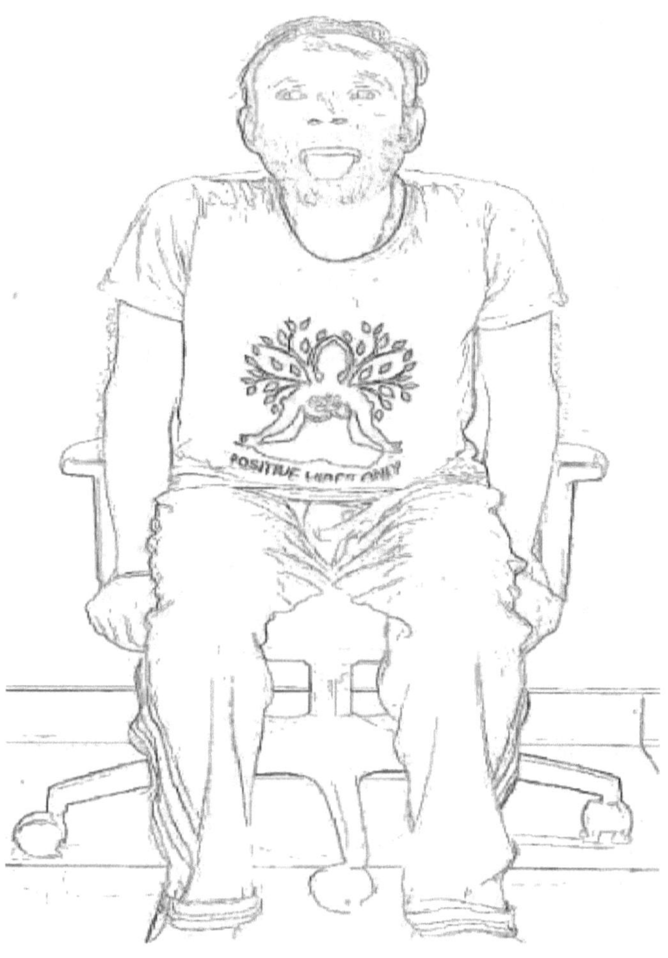

Steps to Perform:

1. Sit comfortably on a sturdy chair with your feet flat on the ground, hip-width apart.
2. Inhale deeply, lifting your arms overhead while lengthening your spine.
3. Exhale slowly, bending forward from the hips and placing your hands on your thighs or the edge of the chair, or a desk in front of you.
4. Extend your arms and spine, keeping your back straight and chest open.
5. Take your tongue out as much possible.

6. Take slow, deep breaths, expanding your ribcage with each inhale and softening your torso with each exhale.
7. Then breath pumping from abdomen. Similar to dog breath.
8. Practice for 20/30 seconds, then slowly return to normal position.

Benefits:
Software engineers spend long hours sitting and working on screens, leading to poor posture, stiffness, and stress. The Seated Dog Breathing (Chair Variation) is a simple yet effective yoga pose that helps counteract these effects.

1. Improves Posture & Reduces Back Pain
Stretches the spine, shoulders, and lower back, counteracting the hunching posture from prolonged sitting. Reduces tension in the lumbar region, preventing chronic back pain.
2. Enhances Lung Capacity & Deep Breathing
Encourages diaphragmatic breathing, improving oxygen flow to the brain and body.
Helps in reducing shallow chest breathing caused by stress and prolonged sitting.
3. Relieves Neck & Shoulder Tension
Opens up the chest and shoulders, reducing stiffness from long hours of typing and using a mouse. Alleviates neck strain caused by forward head posture.
4. Boosts Focus & Mental Clarity
Improves blood circulation, delivering more oxygen to the brain. Helps in reducing fatigue and increasing concentration during coding sessions.
5. Reduces Stress & Anxiety
Activates the parasympathetic nervous system, inducing relaxation. Aids in calming the mind, making it easier to handle work pressure.
6. Increases Energy Levels
Combats sluggishness by improving circulation and releasing endorphins.
Acts as a quick energy booster without needing caffeine.

Bhastrika Pranayama

Bhastrika Pranayama, also known as Bellows Breath, is a powerful and energizing breathing technique that can help IT professionals combat fatigue, mental fog, and stress caused by long hours at a desk. This practice helps to boost energy levels, clear the mind, and improve overall respiratory health.

How Bhastrika Works:
- Quick, rhythmic inhalations and exhalations increase the oxygen supply to the brain and body.
- The forceful breath stimulates the sympathetic nervous system, providing a natural energy boost.
- It mimics the action of a bellows (hence the name), fanning the internal fire (energy) and clearing away mental and physical stagnation.

Practice Bhastrika Pranayama:
1. Starting Position:
   - Sit comfortably with your back straight on a chair or on the floor.
   - Place your hands on your knees in Chin/Gyan Mudra (thumb and index finger touching).
   - Relax your shoulders and close your eyes.
2. Breathing Technique:
   - Inhale deeply, through your nose, expanding your belly and fill the lungs.
   - After full inhalation Exhale forcefully and quickly through your nose making hissing sound, contracting your belly.
   - Inhale deeply and exhale completely.
   - Gradually increase your rapidity of inhale and exhale.
   - Both inhalation and exhalation should be equal in duration and forceful, with a steady rhythm. In bhastrika the inhale and exhale both will be active and forcefully.

3. Breath Cycle:
     o Perform 10-15 breaths (1 round).
     o Take a short pause to breathe normally.
     o Gradually increase to 2-3 rounds as you get
       comfortable.
4. Duration:
     o Beginners: Start with 1-2 minutes.
     o Advanced: Gradually increase to 3-5 minutes.

Benefits for IT Professionals
  1. Boosts Energy Levels:
        Helps overcome mid-afternoon slumps and general
     fatigue caused by sedentary work.
  2. Clears Mental Fog:
        Improves mental clarity and alertness, enhancing
     productivity and focus.
  3. Relieves Stress and Anxiety:
        Quickly reduces stress and helps calm an
     overstimulated mind.
  4. Improves Lung Capacity:
        Strengthens the respiratory system, enhancing
     breathing efficiency and oxygen intake.
  5. Enhances Mood:
        Releases endorphins, helping to reduce irritability
     and elevate mood.
  6. Detoxifies the Body:
        Increases oxygenation, which aids in clearing out
     toxins. It helps in the sinus, bronchitis, and other
     respiratory issues.
  7. Reduces Sleepiness:
        A great alternative to caffeine when you feel
     drowsy during work.

  8. Can helpful for curing the health ailments like asthma,
     headache, migraine, neurological problems and throat
     infection.

Precautions:

1. Avoid if You Have:
    o   High blood pressure
    o   Heart issues
    o   Epilepsy
    o   Major respiratory conditions.
    o   Pregnancy
2. Listen to Your Body:
    o   Stop immediately if you feel dizzy, light-headed, or experience discomfort.
    o   Always practice on an empty stomach or at least 2 hours after a meal.

When to Practice:
*   Morning: To kickstart your day with energy and focus.

Kapalabhati Pranayama

Kapalabhati Pranayama is a powerful breathing technique that offers quick rejuvenation for the mind and body, making it an excellent tool for working professionals, especially those in the IT sector who face long hours of mental strain, screen fatigue, and sedentary work.

Kapalabhati literally translates to 'shining forehead,' and this is precisely what happens with regular practice of this pranayama - a forehead that glows not just on the outside, but also an intellect that becomes sharp and refined.

It symbolizes the clarity, brightness, and focus it brings to the mind.
Practice:

1. Starting Position:
Sit comfortably in a chair with a straight spine, feet flat on the floor, and hands resting on your thighs.
Keep your shoulders relaxed and your neck upright.
2. Breathing Pattern:

Inhale gently through the nose.
Perform a forceful exhalation by quickly pulling your abdominal muscles inward, pushing the breath out through the nose.
The inhalation is passive and automatic, while the exhalation is active and deliberate.
3. Rhythm:
Start with a slow pace (1 exhalation per second).
Aim for 20–30 rapid exhalations per round.
Gradually increase to 60–100 exhalations per round as you get comfortable.
4. Rounds:
Begin with 2–3 rounds, pausing briefly between rounds.
As you build stamina, you can increase to 5 rounds.

When to Practice:
o   Morning: To kickstart your day with energy and clarity.
o   Midday Break: For a quick reset and to overcome post-lunch sluggishness.
o   After Long Screen Time: To refresh your mind and reduce mental fatigue.

Benefits for IT Professionals
o   Mental Clarity: Clears brain fog and enhances focus, which is crucial for solving complex problems.
o   Energy Boost: Provides an instant burst of energy when feeling tired or sluggish.
o   Stress Reduction: Helps relieve anxiety, stress, and mental tension.
o   Detoxification: Cleanses the lungs, sinuses, and respiratory system by expelling toxins.
o   Improves Circulation: Increases oxygen supply to the brain and body.
o   Combats Sedentary Fatigue: Activates abdominal muscles and diaphragm, aiding digestion and reducing bloating.

Precautions:
Not Recommended If You Have:
    o   High blood pressure

- o Heart problems
- o Recent abdominal surgery
- o Severe respiratory issues (e.g., asthma, COPD)
- o Pregnancy or menstruation

Avoid Overdoing It:
- o Start slowly and stop if you feel dizzy or lightheaded.

Ujjayi Pranayama:

Ujjayi Pranayama, also known as "Ocean Breath" or "Victorious Breath," is a calming and balancing breathing technique often used in yoga practice and meditation. For IT professionals who face constant mental demands, screen fatigue, and stressful work environments, incorporating Ujjayi Breath can help restore balance, focus, and calm.

"Uj" = To expand or conquer

"Jaya" = Victory

That's why, Ujjayi is translated as "Victorious Breath" because of its ability to create a sense of empowerment and mastery over the mind and body.

It is often referred to as "Ocean Breath" because the sound produced resembles the rhythmic sound of ocean waves.

Practice Ujjayi Breath

1. Starting Position:
- o Sit comfortably in your chair with a straight spine, feet flat on the floor, and shoulders relaxed.
- o Rest your hand on knee or thigh with Chin/Gyan mudra.
- o Alternatively, you can stand or sit cross-legged if space allows.
2. Breathing Process:
- o Inhale slowly through the nose, Ujjayi pranayama involves partial closure of glottis when inhaling and exhaling by slightly constricting the back of your throat (as if you're trying to fog up a mirror with your breath).

- o You should hear a soft, whisper-like sound, similar to the sound of the ocean waves.
- o Exhale slowly through the nose while maintaining the same throat constriction and gentle sound.
3. Rhythm:
- o Make your inhalation and exhalation equal in length.
- o Aim for 4–6 seconds for each inhale and exhale.
- o Gradually increase the duration as you become more comfortable.
4. Duration:
- o Start with 2–5 minutes of Ujjayi Breath.
- o As you become familiar, extend to 10 minutes or integrate it into longer meditation sessions.

Benefits of Ujjayi for IT Professionals
1. Reduces Stress and Anxiety: Helps activate the parasympathetic nervous system, reducing stress levels and promoting relaxation.
2. Increases Focus and Concentration: The rhythmic sound and breath pattern help anchor attention, enhancing mental clarity.
3. Relieves Fatigue: Counteracts the exhaustion caused by long hours of work, boosting overall energy levels.
4. Improves Posture Awareness: Encourages deep diaphragmatic breathing, which supports proper posture.
5. Regulates Emotions: Helps manage emotional turbulence, making it easier to respond calmly to challenges.
6. Promotes Mindfulness: The audible breath creates an anchor for mindfulness during work breaks or meditation.
7. Reduces Eye Strain: Relaxing the mind indirectly helps relieve eye strain from prolonged screen time.

Tips for Practicing Ujjayi at Your Desk
1. Take Regular Breaks: Incorporate Ujjayi breathing during short breaks to reset your mind.
2. Close Your Eyes (Optional): Closing your eyes helps deepen relaxation, but you can keep them open if needed.

3. Focus on the Sound: The ocean-like sound helps you stay anchored and mindful.
4. Combine with a Mudra:
    o Chin Mudra (thumb and index finger touching) for focus.
    o Shuni Mudra (thumb and middle finger touching) for patience and discipline.
5. Maintain Proper Posture: Keep your spine straight to allow full, deep breaths.

Bhramari Pranayama (Bee Breath):

Bhramari, derived from the Sanskrit word Bhramara (the black Indian humming bee called Bhramari), is a calming breathing technique that involves making a soft, humming sound, similar to humming bee during exhalation. This technique resembles the sound of a buzzing bee and helps quiet the mind, reduce mental stress, release frustration, anger and improve focus.

Why is Bhramari for IT Professionals?
IT professionals often experience:
    o Mental fatigue from prolonged cognitive work.
    o Anxiety and stress due to tight deadlines and high expectations.
    o Lack of focus caused by multitasking and distractions.
    o Sleep disturbances due to extended screen time and irregular work hours.
Bhramari Pranayama benefits:
    o Calming the nervous system and reducing anxiety.
    o Improving concentration and mental clarity.
    o Releasing tension in the forehead and head region.
    o Mental Clarity: Clears mental fog and improves cognitive function.
    o Stress Relief: Reduces anxiety and induces relaxation.
    o Better Sleep: Helps ease the mind before bedtime.
    o Enhanced Focus: Increases attention span during work tasks.

- o Breathing Awareness: Improves lung function and breath control.
- o Speed up the healing of tear tissue.
- o Cure hypertension and depression.

Practice Bhramari Pranayama:

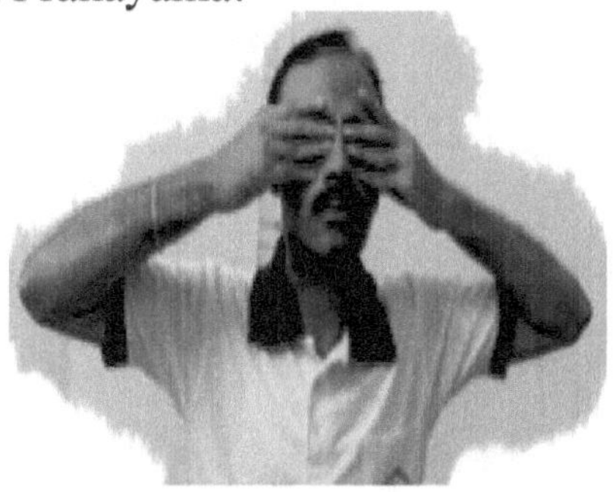

1. Posture:

- Sit comfortably in a chair or on the floor.
- Keep your back straight, shoulders relaxed, and feet flat on the ground if seated on a chair.

2. Hand Placement:

- Close your eyes gently.
- Place your thumbs on the cartilage of your ears (the flap that can close the ear canal).
- Lightly rest your index fingers slightly above on your eyebrow.
- Let your middle on eyelids, ring finger on your nostril, and little fingers above the lips.
- Fold the tongue and touch the upper palate with the tip of tongue. Keep the lips closed and upper set of teeth and lower set of teeth should not touch. (Initially you can practice without this step. Simply keep lips close and practice.)

3. Breathing:

- Take a deep breath in through your nose, filling your lungs completely.
- As you exhale, press lightly on the ear cartilage and produce a low, steady humming sound like a buzzing bee ("hmmm").
- Feel the vibration in your head, especially around your forehead and sinuses.

4. Duration:

- Continue this process for 5-7 rounds. Each round should last about 15-20 seconds.
- After the final round, sit in silence for a minute and observe the calmness.

When to Practice Bhramari

- During Work Breaks: For quick stress relief or when feeling overwhelmed.
- Before Sleep: To wind down after a long day.
- Can be practice anytime of the day

Contraindications:
If you are feeling dizzy when practicing stop the exercise and start normal breathing.
Avoid when having a severe ear infection or ear pain.
Careful when migraine pain is active.

Sheetali Pranayama (Cooling Pranayama):

Sheetali is derived from the Sanskrit word Sheetal, meaning "cooling" or "soothing." This pranayama helps cool down the body, calm the mind, and reduce stress and anxiety. By regulating body temperature and calming the nervous system, Sheetali Pranayama acts as a mental and physical reset, ideal for busy IT professionals.

Why is Sheetali Beneficial for IT Professionals?

IT professionals often experience:
o Mental Overload: Long hours of problem-solving and coding lead to cognitive fatigue.
o Screen Fatigue: Continuous exposure to screens can strain the eyes and increase body heat.
o Stress and Irritability: Tight deadlines and multitasking can spike stress levels.
o Poor Sleep Quality: Work-related anxiety can disturb sleep patterns.

Sheetali Pranayama can helps by:

o Cooling the Body: Reduces internal body heat, alleviating physical tension.
o Relaxing the Mind: Soothes the nervous system and reduces stress.
o Promoting Calmness: Helps lower anxiety and enhances focus.
o Cools the Body: Quickly reduces body heat from mental stress or screen exposure.
o Relieves Stress: Calms the nervous system, reducing anxiety and irritability, also this have positive impact on endocrine gland and helps to keep blood pressure lowered.
o Reduces Eye Strain: Provides relief from dry eyes, headaches, and screen fatigue.
o Promotes Better Sleep: Prepares the mind and body for restful sleep.
o Refreshes the mind for enhanced concentration.
o Sheetali pranayama gives control over hunger and thirst.

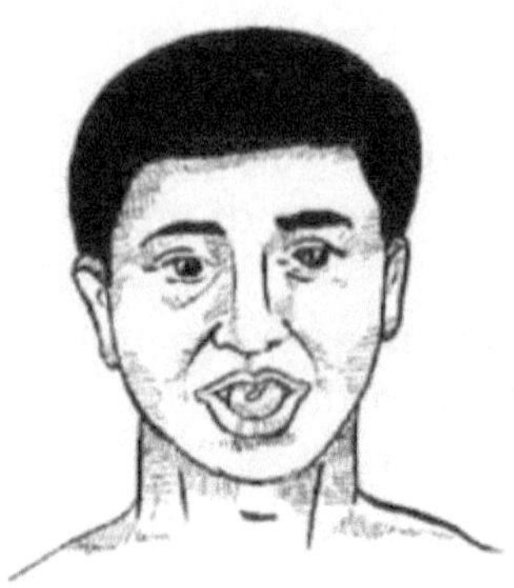

Practice:

1. Posture:
   - Sit comfortably in a chair or on the floor with your back straight.
   - Rest your hands on your knees and close your eyes gently.
2. Hand Placement:
   - Place your hands on your knees or in Chin.
3. Tongue Position:
   - Take your tongue slightly forward and Roll your tongue lengthwise into a tube shape by curling the sides of the tongue upward.
4. Breathing:
   - Inhale Slowly: Take a deep breath in through the rolled tongue.
   - Feel the cool air entering your mouth and filling your lungs.
   - Close Your Mouth: After a full inhale, close your mouth and exhale slowly through your nose.
5. Focus:
   - Focus on the sensation of coolness during the inhale and relaxation during the exhale.
6. Duration:
   - Repeat the process for 5-10 rounds or for 3-5 minutes.
7. After Practice:

    o Sit quietly with normal breathing for a minute to experience the calming effects.

When to Practice Sheetali

- During Work Breaks: To refresh your mind and reduce heat or frustration.
- After Long Screen Time: To ease eye strain and mental fatigue.
- Before Bed: To cool down your system and prepare for sleep.
- After Intense Work Sessions: To calm down after solving complex problems.

Precautions:

Avoid If You Have:

- Low Blood Pressure: The cooling effect may cause further drops in blood pressure.
- Respiratory Issues: Severe asthma, bronchitis, or congestion may make it difficult to inhale through the mouth.
- Cold or Cough: Inhaling cool air can worsen cold symptoms.
- Sensitivity to Cold: If you feel discomfort due to cold sensitivity, avoid this practice.

Avoid Practicing in Cold Weather:
If the environment is already cold, this practice may lead to discomfort or chills.

Empty Stomach: Practice at least 2-3 hours after a meal for the best results.

Sheetkari Pranayama (Hissing Breath):

Sheetkari comes from the Sanskrit word Sheet meaning "cooling," and Kari meaning "producing." In this practice, a hissing sound is created while inhaling through the teeth, bringing a cooling effect to the body and mind.

Why is Sheetkari Beneficial for IT Professionals?

IT professionals often face:

- Cognitive Overload: Long hours of mental work lead to fatigue.
- Stress and Anxiety: Deadlines, debugging, and multitasking increase anxiety.
- Eye Strain: Extended screen exposure causes dry eyes, headaches, and tension.
- Increased Body Heat: Sedentary work and stress raise internal body heat.
- Sleep Disturbances: Overactive minds and late hours disrupt restful sleep.

Sheetkari Pranayama helps by:

- Cooling the Body and Mind: Reduces heat-related discomfort and irritability.
- Relieving Eye Strain: Refreshes the eyes and alleviates headaches. Provides relief from dry eyes.
- Calming the Nervous System: Reduces mental stress and anxiety.
- Promoting Mental Clarity: Improves focus and cognitive function. Clears mental fog, enhancing clarity and concentration.
- Enhancing Sleep Quality: Prepares the body and mind for relaxation and sleep.
- Relieves Stress: Calms the mind, reducing anxiety and mental fatigue.
- Promotes Relaxation: Helps unwind before bed or after a stressful task.

When to Practice Sheetkari

- o During Work Breaks: To reset your mind and reduce stress.
- o After Long Screen Sessions: To ease eye strain and headaches.
- o Before Bedtime: To cool down after a stressful day and promote sleep.

Practice:

1. Posture:
   - o Sit comfortably in a chair or on the floor with your back straight.
   - o Rest your hands on your knees with Chin Mudra.
   - o Close your eyes gently.
2. Hand Placement:
   - o Keep your hands relaxed on your knees or thighs.
3. Teeth Position:
   - o Fold the tip of the tongue inwards horizontally. Folded tongue should come slightly out between the two rows of teeth keeping narrow opening on both sides.
   - o Separate your lips slightly to expose your teeth.
4. Breathing:
   - o Inhale Slowly: Breathe in deeply through the both side, producing a soft hissing sound (like a gentle "hhissss").
   - o Feel the cool air moving over your tongue and into your lungs.
   - o Exhale Through the Nose: Close your mouth and exhale slowly through your nose.
5. Focus:
   - o Pay attention to the sensation of coolness during the inhale and the relaxation during the exhale.
   - o Allow your mind to settle with each breath.
6. Duration:
   - o Repeat for 5-10 rounds or for about 3-5 minutes.

7. After Practice:
   o   Sit quietly with your eyes closed and take a few normal
       breaths, enjoying the sense of calm.

Time Required: 5-7 minutes.

Precautions:

1. Avoid If You Have:
   o   Low Blood Pressure: The cooling effect may further lower
       your blood pressure, causing dizziness.
   o   Respiratory Issues: Severe asthma, bronchitis, or nasal
       congestion may make this practice difficult.
   o   Tooth Sensitivity: If your teeth are sensitive to cold air,
       this practice may cause discomfort.
   o   Cold or Cough: Inhaling cool air may aggravate
       symptoms.
2. Avoid in Cold Weather:
   o   If the environment is already cold, practicing Sheetkari
       may cause chills or discomfort.
3. Empty Stomach:
   o   Practice at least 2-3 hours after a meal to avoid discomfort.

Sadanta Pranayama:

Sadanta means "through the teeth" in Sanskrit. This
pranayama is a cooling breath practice where air is drawn in
through the teeth and exhaled through the nose. Like Sheetali and
Sheetkari, it helps reduce internal heat, calm the mind, and refresh
the body.

Why is Sadanta Beneficial for IT Professionals?

IT professionals often deal with:

•   Mental Exhaustion: Prolonged cognitive tasks lead to brain
    fatigue.

- Stress and Anxiety: Coding errors, deadlines, and multitasking create mental strain.
- Eye Strain: Staring at screens for extended periods causes dry eyes and headaches.
- Increased Body Heat: Sedentary work, stress, and lack of movement can increase internal heat.
- Frustration and Irritability: Pressure and problem-solving demands can affect mood.

Sadanta Pranayama helps by:

- Cooling the Body: Reduces internal heat and alleviates irritability.
- Soothing the Mind: Calms anxiety and stress, promoting mental clarity.
- Easing Frustration: Helps manage emotions and improves mood.
- Improving Sleep Quality: Prepares the mind for restful sleep after a stressful day.
- Relieves Stress and Anxiety: Calms the nervous system and promotes relaxation.
- Eases Eye Strain: Helps relieve headaches and tension caused by screen use.
- Enhances Focus: Clears mental fog and improves concentration.
- Promotes Emotional Balance: Reduces frustration and irritability.

When to Practice Sadanta

- During Breaks: To refresh the mind and body after intense work sessions.
- After Screen Time: To relieve eye strain and reduce tension.
- Before Bedtime: To cool down and prepare for sleep.
- After Intense Mental Work: To clear mental clutter and reset.

Practice:

1. Posture:
   o Sit comfortably on a chair or the floor with your back straight.
   o Rest your hands on your knees or thighs, palms facing up with chin mudra.
2. Mouth and Teeth Position:
   o Gently touch your upper and lower teeth together.
   o Keep your lips slightly parted so that your teeth are exposed.
3. Inhale Through the Teeth:
   o Inhale slowly and deeply through the gaps(through the crevices of the teeth) between your teeth. And continuously into the mouth and passing down the throat into lungs.
   o You may hear a soft, hissing sound as the cool air flows in.
4. Exhale Through the Nose:
   o Close your mouth and exhale slowly and completely through your nose.
   o Focus on releasing tension with each exhale.
5. Focus:
   o Concentrate on the cool sensation during the inhale and the sense of relaxation during the exhale.
6. Duration:
   o Practice for 5-10 rounds or for 3-5 minutes.
   o After the final round, sit quietly and breathe normally for a minute.

Time Required: 5-7 minutes.

Precautions:

1. Avoid If You Have:
   o Low Blood Pressure: The cooling effect may lower blood pressure further, causing dizziness.
   o Cold, Cough, or Congestion: Inhaling cool air may worsen respiratory issues.

- o   Sensitive Teeth: The practice may cause discomfort for those with dental sensitivity.
2. Avoid in Cold Weather:
- o   Practicing in a cold environment may lead to chills or discomfort.
3. Empty Stomach:
- o   Practice on an empty stomach or at least 2-3 hours after a meal for the best results.

Chandra Nadi Pranayama (Left Nostril Breathing):

Chandra Nadi refers to the "Moon Channel" in yogic philosophy, associated with the left nostril and the ida nadi, which represents cooling, calming, and introspective energy. Pranayama, or breath control, regulates the flow of energy through this channel, promoting relaxation and emotional stability.

For IT professionals dealing with high-pressure situations, Chandra Nadi Pranayama is an excellent tool for calming the mind, reducing stress, and regaining focus.

Why is Chandra Nadi Pranayama Beneficial for IT Professionals?

IT professionals face challenges like:

- Stress and Anxiety: Deadlines, multitasking, and complex problem-solving.
- Mental Fatigue: Prolonged screen time and cognitive overload.
- Emotional Imbalance: Frustration, irritability, and burnout.
- Sleep Issues: Work-related thoughts interfering with restful sleep.

Benefits of Chandra Nadi Pranayama:

- Calms the Mind: Activates the parasympathetic nervous system, reducing stress and anxiety.
- Promotes Relaxation: Provides a sense of inner calm and emotional balance.
- Improves Mental Clarity: Enhances focus and concentration.
- Aids Sleep: Helps the mind unwind, supporting better sleep quality.
- Balances Emotions: Reduces frustration and promotes patience.
- Cools the Body: Alleviates internal heat and tension.

When to Practice Chandra Nadi Pranayama

- During Work Breaks: To reset the mind and reduce stress.
- During Emotional Upsets: To regain balance and calmness.
- After Intense Cognitive Tasks: To recharge mental energy.

Practice Chandra Nadi Pranayama

Step-by-Step Instructions

1. Posture:
   o Sit comfortably on a chair or the floor with your back straight.
   o Rest your hands on your knees or thighs, palms facing up.
2. Hand Position (Vishnu Mudra):
   o Fold the index and middle fingers of your right hand toward the palm.
   o Use your right thumb to close your right nostril and your ring finger to close the left nostril as needed.
3. Begin the Practice:
   o Close the Right Nostril: Gently press your right thumb against your right nostril, closing it completely.
   o Inhale Through the Left Nostril: Breathe in slowly and deeply through your left nostril, filling your lungs with air.
   o Exhale Through the Left Nostril: Continue to keep the right nostril closed and exhale slowly through the left nostril.

4. Focus on the Breath:
   o Pay attention to the cool sensation of the air as it enters and exits through your left nostril.
   o Feel the calming effect spreading through your body with each breath.
5. Duration:
   o Repeat for 5-10 minutes or for 10-20 cycles.
   o Gradually increase the duration as you become more comfortable.
6. End the Practice:
   o Lower your hand, take a few normal breaths, and notice the sense of relaxation.

Precautions:

1. Avoid If You Have:
   o Respiratory Issues: Severe nasal congestion, sinus infections, or difficulty breathing.
   o Low Energy Levels: Practicing Chandra Nadi excessively during the day may make you too relaxed or drowsy.
2. Practice in a Calm Environment:
   o Ensure you are in a quiet, comfortable place without distractions.
3. Avoid Cold Environments:
   o Practicing in very cold weather or air-conditioned spaces for long periods may cause discomfort.
4. Empty Stomach:
   o Perform on an empty stomach or at least 2-3 hours after a meal.

Tips for Effective Practice

1. Consistency is Key:
   o Practice daily, even for just 5 minutes, to experience lasting benefits.
2. Focus on the Breath:
   o Keep your mind anchored to the sensation of the breath to deepen the calming effect.

3. Combine with Mindfulness:
    o   Pair with a short mindfulness meditation for holistic
        relaxation.

Surya Nadi Pranayama (Right Nostril Breathing):

Surya Nadi refers to the "Sun Channel" in yogic philosophy,
associated with the right nostril and the pingala nadi, which
represents heat, energy, and vitality. This pranayama technique
activates the right nostril to stimulate energy flow, increase
alertness, and promote productivity.

For IT professionals, Surya Nadi Pranayama can enhance focus
and provide a mental boost during sluggish mornings or moments
of mental fatigue.

Why is Surya Nadi Pranayama Beneficial for IT Professionals?

IT professionals often experience:

- Mental Fatigue: Long hours of coding and debugging.
- Low Energy Levels: Lack of physical activity and
  sedentary work.
- Difficulty Concentrating: Distractions and workload stress.
- Morning Sluggishness: Lack of motivation or energy to
  start the day.

Benefits of Surya Nadi Pranayama:

- Boosts Energy: Stimulates the nervous system and
  combats lethargy.
- Enhances Focus: Improves cognitive function and mental
  clarity.
- Promotes Warmth: Increases internal heat, improving
  circulation and vitality.

- Improves Mood: Alleviates feelings of laziness or low energy.
- Increases Productivity: Sharpens mental faculties for high-performance tasks.

When to Practice Surya Nadi Pranayama

- In the Morning: To energize the body and prepare for the day.
- Before Work: To boost focus and motivation.
- During Low Energy Moments: Midday slumps or post-lunch drowsiness.
- Before Intense Cognitive Tasks: Coding sessions, problem-solving, or presentations.

How to Practice Surya Nadi Pranayama

Step-by-Step Instructions

1. Posture:
   o Sit in a comfortable position with your back straight and shoulders relaxed.
   o Rest your hands on your knees or thighs, palms facing up.
2. Hand Position (Vishnu Mudra):
   o Use your right hand, folding the index and middle fingers toward the palm.
   o Use the right thumb to close the right nostril and the ring finger to close the left nostril as needed.
3. Begin the Practice:
   o Close the Left Nostril: Gently press your ring finger against your left nostril to close it.
   o Inhale Through the Right Nostril: Take a deep, slow breath in through your right nostril.
   o Exhale Through the Right Nostril: Continue to keep the left nostril closed and exhale slowly through the right nostril.
4. Focus on the Breath:
   o Pay attention to the warmth and energy of the air as it flows in and out of your right nostril.

- o   Feel the energizing effect spreading through your body.
5. Duration:
- o   Start with 5 minutes or 10-20 cycles. Gradually increase to 10-15 minutes as you feel comfortable.
6. End the Practice:
- o   Lower your hand, take a few normal breaths, and notice the increased energy and focus.

Precautions

Avoid If You Have:

- o   High Blood Pressure: The energizing effect may exacerbate symptoms.
- o   Fever: The heating nature may increase body temperature.
- o   Hyperactivity or Anxiety: May overstimulate an already overactive mind.
2. Practice in Moderation:
- o   Avoid over-practicing as it may lead to restlessness or imbalance.
3. Empty Stomach:
- o   Perform on an empty stomach or at least 2-3 hours after a meal.

Tips for Effective Practice

1. Practice in the Morning:
- o   Start your day with 5-10 minutes of Surya Nadi Pranayama for an energetic boost.
2. Combine with Light Movement:
- o   Pair with gentle stretches or a short yoga routine to awaken the body fully.
3. Focus on Intentions:
- o   Set an intention for your day as you practice, such as productivity, focus, or positivity.
4. Maintain a Straight Posture:
- o   Keep your spine aligned for optimal energy flow.

Surya Nadi vs. Chandra Nadi

Aspect	Surya Nadi (Right Nostril)	Chandra Nadi (Left Nostril)
Associated Energy	Heating, energizing, masculine	Cooling, calming, feminine
Time of Practice	Morning or during low energy	Evening or during stress
Effect	Boosts energy and focus	Promotes relaxation and calmness

Dog Breathing(Panting Breath):

Dog Breathing is a pranayama technique that involves fast, shallow breathing through the mouth, mimicking the panting of a dog. It is known for its energizing and detoxifying effects, making it a great option for quick stress relief and mental clarity.

For IT professionals, who often face physical and mental fatigue due to prolonged sitting and screen exposure, Dog Breathing provides a quick way to recharge energy and reduce stress.

Why is Dog Breathing Beneficial for IT Professionals?

IT professionals often experience:

- Stress and Anxiety: Tight deadlines, multitasking, and high-pressure work environments.
- Mental Exhaustion: Long hours of problem-solving and coding.
- Physical Tension: Stiffness from prolonged desk work.

Benefits of Dog Breathing:

- Releases Stress: Quickly alleviates tension from prolonged sitting or intense tasks and mental fatigue.

- Boosts Energy: Activates the body's natural energy reserves.
- Improves Focus: Clears mental fog, enhancing concentration.
- Detoxifies the Body: Promotes the release of toxins through increased oxygenation.
- Strengthens Respiratory System: Improves lung capacity and breath control.
- Instant Energy Boost: Quickly revitalizes the mind and body.
- Mental Clarity: Clears the mind for better problem-solving and focus.

- Breath Awareness: Enhances overall respiratory health.
- Quick Relaxation: Helps calm the nervous system in just a few moments.

When to Practice Dog Breathing

- During Short Breaks: To relieve stress and re-energize.
- After Intense Work Sessions: To release tension and relax.
- In the Afternoon: To counteract the midday energy slump.

How to Practice Dog Breathing

Step-by-Step Instructions

1. Posture:
   o Sit comfortably on a chair or the floor with your back straight.
   o Place your hands on your thighs or knees for support.
2. Mouth Position:
   o Open your mouth slightly, sticking your tongue out slightly like a panting dog.
3. Breathing:
   o Rapidly inhale and exhale through your mouth in short, shallow breaths, mimicking a dog's panting.
   o Keep the rhythm steady and consistent.
4. Duration:

- o Begin with 15-30 seconds of panting.
- o Gradually increase to 1-2 minutes as you build stamina.
5. Focus:
- o Keep your mind focused on the sensation of breath moving through your mouth and the cooling effect on your body.
6. End the Practice:
- o Close your mouth and return to normal nasal breathing.
- o Take a few deep breaths through your nose to relax.

Precautions

Avoid If You Have:

- o Respiratory Issues: Severe asthma, bronchitis, or chronic obstructive pulmonary disease (COPD).
- o High Blood Pressure: Rapid breathing may temporarily increase heart rate.
- o Dizziness: If you feel lightheaded, stop the practice immediately.
2. Practice in Moderation:
- o Avoid overdoing the technique, as it may lead to hyperventilation.
3. Comfortable Environment:
- o Perform in a quiet, calm space to focus fully on your breath.

Tips for Effective Practice

1. Combine with Gentle Stretches:
- o Pair Dog Breathing with light neck and shoulder stretches to relieve tension further.
2. Practice with an Open Mind:
- o Embrace the playful nature of the technique to make it more enjoyable and effective.
3. Stay Hydrated:
- o Drink water before practice to prevent dryness in the mouth.
4. Morning or Midday:

o   Best practiced when you need a quick boost of energy or
    clarity.

Nadi Shodhana Pranayama:

Nadi Shodhana Pranayama, also known as "Alternate
Nostril Breathing," is a powerful yogic breathing technique that
helps to balance the flow of energy in the body and calm the mind.
The word Nadi means "channel" or "flow," and Shodhana means
"purification" or "cleansing." This practice is designed to purify
the energy channels (Nadis) in the body and promote mental
clarity, relaxation, and physical health.

Why Nadi Shodhana is Beneficial for IT Professionals

1. Stress Relief and Relaxation:
    o   IT professionals often work under high-pressure deadlines
        and demanding workloads. Nadi Shodhana helps activate
        the parasympathetic nervous system, which induces
        relaxation, lowers stress, and calms the mind.
2. Enhanced Focus and Mental Clarity:
    o   Alternating nostril breathing balances the left and right
        hemispheres of the brain, improving cognitive function,
        memory, and concentration. This can lead to better
        productivity in tasks like coding, debugging, or problem-
        solving.
3. Improved Energy and Reduced Fatigue:
    o   Prolonged desk work can cause physical exhaustion and
        mental burnout. Nadi Shodhana revitalizes the body by
        enhancing oxygen flow and balancing energy levels,
        making it an effective midday refresh.
4. Emotional Balance and Burnout Prevention:
    o   Regular practice helps regulate emotions, reducing
        frustration, irritability, and the risk of burnout often
        associated with long hours and challenging tasks in the IT
        sector.
5. Creativity Boost:

o   This pranayama enhances mental calmness and balance, fostering an environment for creative thinking—critical for solving complex problems or brainstorming innovative solutions.

6. Better Sleep Quality:
    o   The calming effects of Nadi Shodhana promote restful sleep, which is essential for recovery and maintaining high performance during work hours.

How to Practice Nadi Shodhana Pranayama as an IT Professional:

1. Create a Comfortable Space:
    o   Find a quiet place at home or work where you can practice undisturbed. You can perform this pranayama at your desk or in a break room, but ensure you're seated comfortably with your back straight and shoulders relaxed.
2. Posture:
    o   Sit in a comfortable cross-legged position on the floor or sit upright on a chair with your feet flat on the ground. Keep your spine straight, shoulders relaxed, and hands resting gently on your knees.
3. Use the Vishnu Mudra:
    o   Bring your right hand up to your face. Fold the index and middle fingers down toward your palm. Use your thumb to close the right nostril and your ring finger to close the left nostril.
4. Begin the Practice:
    o   Close your right nostril and inhale deeply through your left nostril, focusing on slow, steady breaths.
    o   Close your left nostril with your ring finger, then release your right nostril and exhale through the right nostril slowly.
    o   Inhale through the right nostril, then close the right nostril and exhale through the left nostril.
    o   This completes one cycle. Continue for 5-10 minutes, gradually increasing the duration as you become more comfortable.
5. Frequency:

o   Begin with 5 minutes of practice, once or twice a day. You can gradually increase the time to 10-15 minutes as you build comfort with the practice.

6. Timing:

o   The best time to practice Nadi Shodhana is early in the morning, after waking up, or in the evening to unwind before bed. However, IT professionals can also practice it during work breaks, especially when feeling stressed or fatigued.

Chapter 5

Mudra chair variations

Mudras

Mudra(मुद्रा) is a Sanskrit word and meaning in English as like 'Seal/Gesture/Sign'. मुद्रा is a symbolic gesture or position used in yoga, meditation. According to Bharat's yogic philosophy, मुद्रा balance the energy flow within the body. It's balance the five elements in the body.
So मुद्रा enhance the physical, mental and emotional well-being.

Five fingers to balance the five elements:
Thumb .... Fire
Index........... Air
Middle......... Sky/Space
Ring............ Earth
Little........... Water

Before we explore the transformative power of mudras, let us set an intention for peace, well-being, and fulfilment for ourselves and others.

"ॐ सर्वेषां स्वस्तिर्भवतु ।"

"May there be well-being for all."

"सर्वेषां शान्तिर्भवतु ।"

"May there be peace for all."

"सर्वेषां पूर्णंभवतु ।"

"May there be fulfillment for all."

"सर्वेषां मङ्गलंभवतु ।"

"May there be auspiciousness for all."

"ॐ शान्तिः शान्तिः शान्तिः ॥"

"Om, peace, peace, peace."

Chin mudra:

Chin Mudra is a widely used hand gesture in pranayama and meditation. It brings back your consciousness.

Why IT Employees Benefit from Chin Mudra

- o Reduces mental fatigue from long hours of screen time.
- o Enhances focus and creativity by calming the racing thoughts.
- o Eases physical tension caused by prolonged sitting.
- o provide a valuable tool for mental well-being and productivity in a high-pressure work environment.

Quick 3-Minute Breathing Break

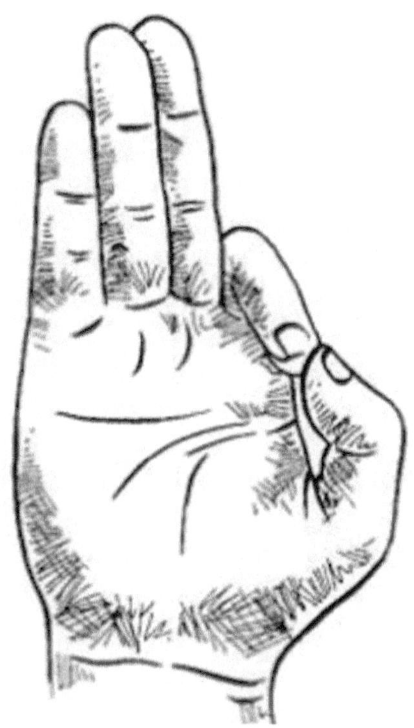

Positions:
- o Sit Upright in your chair with your feet flat on the ground.

Hand positions:
- o Place your hands on your thighs or knees, palms facing downwards.
- o Touch the tip of your thumb and index finger together while keeping the other three fingers extended.

Breathing:
- o Close your eyes, 3 time practice a deep breath in through your nose, and exhale slowly through your mouth.
- o Focus on your breath.
- o After 3 time deep breathing practice; start deep breathing in through nose and slowly exhale through nose only. Exhale should be more than inhale.
- o Practice for 3 minutes.

Gyan Mudra:

This is mudra of Knowledge, it's a Gesture of Knowledge.

Why for IT-Professionals:
- o   Represents the connection to knowledge and wisdom.
- o   The upward-facing palms indicate a receptive attitude toward knowledge and higher awareness.
- o   Enhances focus, concentration, and mental clarity. Especially before analytical tasks or problem-solving.

Positions:

Sit Upright in your chair with your feet flat on the ground.

Hand Positions:
- o   Touch the tip of the thumb and the index finger together, forming a circle.
- o   The other fingers remain extended but relaxed.
- o   Palms face upward when placed on the knees or thighs.

Differences

Aspect	Chin Mudra	Gyan Mudra
Palm Position	Downward-facing	Upward-facing
Symbolism	Consciousness, grounding	Knowledge, receptivity
Use Case	Self-awareness, grounding meditation	Focus, learning, and concentration
Effect	Calms and grounds the mind	Invigorates and stimulates the mind

Hakini Mudra:

In Sanskrit, Hakini means power or rule. This mudra gives the practitioner the power to control their mind. This mudra is useful for those who need mental sharpness and problem-solving abilities, making it ideal for IT professionals and anyone engaged in mentally demanding tasks.

Why Hakini Mudra is Ideal for IT Professionals:

- Improves and deepens the breathing, enables good oxygenation to the brain and hence improves brain functions. And helps to clear the brain fog from long hours of coding and screen time.
- Enhances the memory power
- Improves concentration
- Calms the mind and opens it towards clear thinking
- It is a good gesture for the students, improves their academic performance
- Promotes coordination between the right and left hemispheres of the brain, hence it coordinates creativity and logical thinking
- Promotes clarity of thoughts and hence helps in making proper decisions
- Develops one's connection with the third eye chakra and promotes intuition
- This mudra helps in reducing depression, anxiety and stress.
- It helps balancing blood pressure.

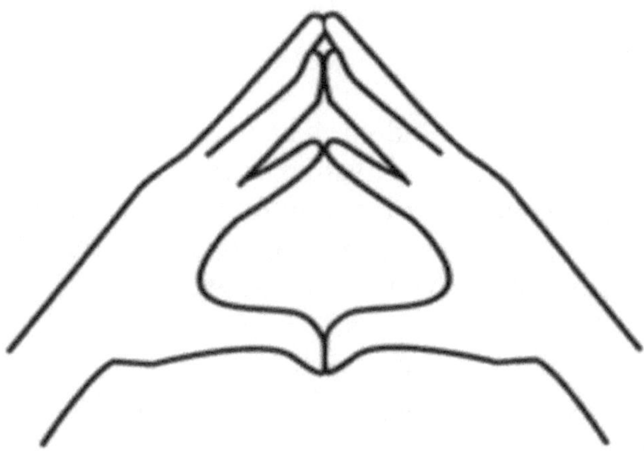

Practice:
- Begin with any comfortable seated posture such as sitting on chair if you are in office, else Padmasana (Lotus Pose), Vajrasana (Thunderbolt Pose), or Sukhasana (Easy Pose).
- Bring your hands in front of your chest with both palms facing each other.

- Gently bring your hands together by joining them at your fingertips.
- Keep your eyes open and gently gaze forward toward agna chakra(Third Eye).
- As you exhale, return your gaze forward.
- You can practice for 3/5 minutes.
- Finally close your eyes and relax.

Additionally to enhance the benefits of this mudra, you can also practice Hakini Mudra as follows.

- Close your eyes and roll them up to set over the third eye chakra as a gaze when inhaling.
- Place your tongue on the soft palate or the roof of the mouth (khechari mudra). Touch the palate when breathing in and release when breathing out.

Uttarabodhi Mudra:

The Uttarabodhi Mudra is a hand gesture associated with awakening inner wisdom, cultivating confidence, and channelling positive energy. This mudra is useful for moments when clarity, focus, or inspiration is needed, making it particularly valuable for IT professionals dealing with mental fatigue or stress.

Why It's Valuable for IT Professionals
- Quick Reset: Easy to practice in short breaks, even while seated at your desk.
- Encourages Positivity: Helps cultivate optimism and resilience during high-pressure works.
- Boosts Productivity: Enhances focus and clarity, which are crucial for analytical and creative tasks.

Benefits of Uttarabodhi Mudra for working professionals:

1. Enhances Confidence:
   o Promotes a sense of empowerment and self-assurance, ideal for boosting morale before meetings or challenging tasks.
2. Improves Focus and Clarity:
   o Helps clear mental clutter, making it easier to concentrate on complex coding or analytical work.
3. Relieves Stress:
   o The hand positioning encourages calm breathing, which aids in reducing anxiety and stress.
4. Cultivates Positive Energy:
   o Supports a mindset of growth and self-awareness, fostering creative solutions to workplace challenges.

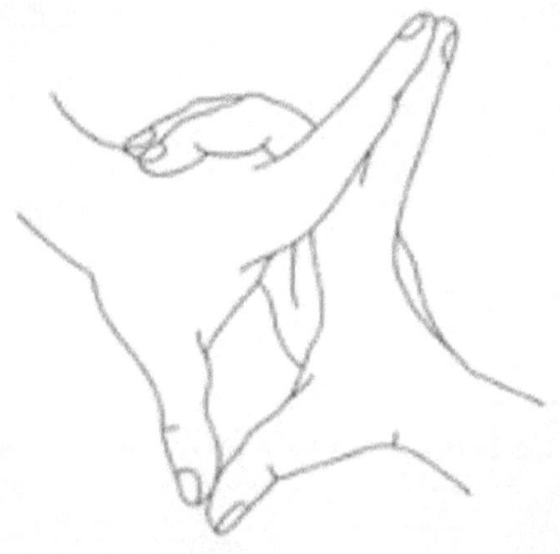

Posture:
- Sit upright in a chair with your feet flat on the ground or in a comfortable seated position.

Hand Position:
- Interlock the fingers of both hands.
- Extend the index fingers, bringing them together to form a point.
- Touch the thumbs lightly together, creating a stable base beneath the index fingers.

Placement:

- Hold the gesture at chest level, just below your heart.
- You can also place your hand at lower abdomen.

Breathing:
- Inhale slowly through your nose, and exhale gently through your nose.
- Focus on maintaining steady, deep breaths for 2-5 minutes.

How to Use Uttarabodhi Mudra During Desk Yoga
1. Morning Mind Reset:
   o Begin your workday by sitting quietly for 3-5 minutes.
   o Form the mudra, close your eyes, and breathe deeply.
   o Set a positive intention, such as: "I am focused and capable."
2. Midday Rejuvenation:
   o When mental fatigue sets in, pause briefly.
   o Hold the mudra, take 5 deep breaths, and visualize light radiating from within.
3. Before Presentations or Meetings:
   o Use this mudra to centre yourself and boost confidence.
   o Focus on steady breathing and remind yourself of your preparedness.

Prana Mudra:
Prana mudra is a mudra or hand gesture which is known for enhancing the vital energy.

Why Prana Mudra is for IT Professionals:
   o Quick & Convenient:
      Can be practiced sitting at a desk without needing to move from your chair. This makes it a perfect choice during short breaks or between tasks.

   o Releases Tension:
      Relieves the tension caused by sitting in the same posture for long hours, allowing for physical and mental relaxation.

o   Accessible and Simple:
    The mudra is easy to learn and requires no special equipment. It can be integrated into daily office routines to increase overall well-being.

o   Promotes Mental and Physical Balance:
    Encourages balance between the mental energy used for problem-solving and physical energy, preventing burnout.

Practice:

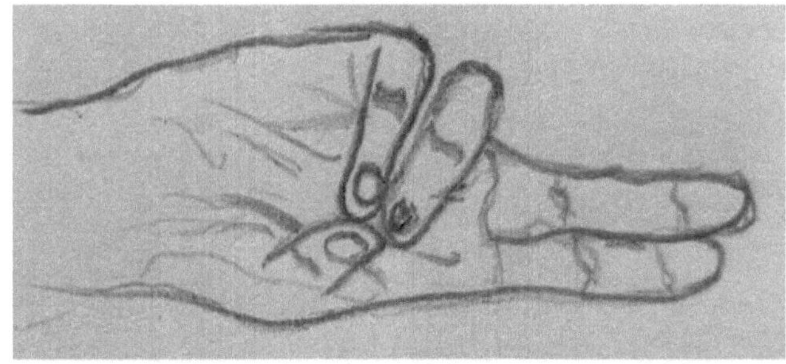

Posture:
- Sit in a comfortable position with your back straight, either on a chair or on the floor.
- Ensure your head is aligned with the spine, and your shoulders are relaxed.

Gesture:
- Touch the tips of the thumb, ring finger, and little finger together.
- Keep the index and middle fingers extended, relaxed, and straight.

Hand Placement:
- Rest your hands on your knees or thighs, with the palms facing upward.

Breathing:
- Focus on slow, deep, and conscious breathing.
- Inhale deeply through your nose and exhale gently through your nose.

- Concentrate on your breathing.

How to Use This During Your Desk Work:
- o Energy Boosting:

  Begin your workday by practicing Prana Mudra for 5 minutes to awaken your body and mind. Take a few deep breaths and set a positive intention for the day ahead, such as: "I am ready for whatever challenges come my way."

- o Refresher:

  After sitting for hours, use this mudra during a quick break, whenever you'll feel low energy, It will recharge your energy levels and relieve mental exhaustion. Close your eyes and take a few deep breaths while practicing this mudra to reset your energy.

- o Post-Work Relaxation:

  Use this mudra as part of your evening routine to release the stress and fatigue accumulated throughout the day. It can be helpful in shifting from work mode to personal time.

Benefits of Prana Mudra for IT Professionals
1. Boosts Energy and Vitality:
   - o Prana Mudra activates the root energy (prana) in the body, helping combat mental fatigue and physical exhaustion, common among IT professionals after prolonged screen/work time.
2. Relieves Stress:
   - o The gesture aids in reducing mental tension and anxiety, promoting a calm and focused state. Lower the stress under pressured worked culture.
3. Improve Immunity:
   - o Regular practice of Prana Mudra can help strengthen the immune system, making it effective in preventing illnesses caused by stress or poor posture during long working hours.
4. Reduces Eye Strain:

- o Practicing this mudra can also be beneficial for reducing eye strain, a common issue among IT professionals due to long hours in front of screens.
5. Improve the Overall Well-Being:
- o By cultivating life force energy, this mudra promotes a sense of vitality, helping you stay energized and engaged throughout your workday.

Shuni Mudra:

Shuni Mudra, is known as the Mudra of Patience, is a hand gesture that encourages focus, patience, and discipline. Shuni means Saturn in Sanskrit. This mudra may strengthening the Solar Plexus, which will boost your willpower, confidence, discipline, and intuition.

Why Shuni Mudra is Ideal for IT Professionals:
- Quick & Easy:
  - o Shuni Mudra can be performed in any seated position, making it perfect for short breaks during desk work.
  - o No special equipment is needed, making it a convenient practice that can be done anywhere.
- Patience in Problem-Solving:
  - o IT professionals often face situations where patience is required, whether debugging code or working through technical problems.
  - o Shuni Mudra helps develop the necessary patience to approach challenges with a calm, disciplined mindset.
- Stress Management:
  - o It's easy to become stressed in the tech industry, but Shuni Mudra helps to balance emotions and relieve tension, ensuring that you can handle high-pressure situations with grace.
- Enhance Communication:
  - o Because Shuni Mudra influences the throat chakra, it enhances communication skills. This is essential for IT professionals who work in teams or need to explain technical issues in a clear, concise manner.

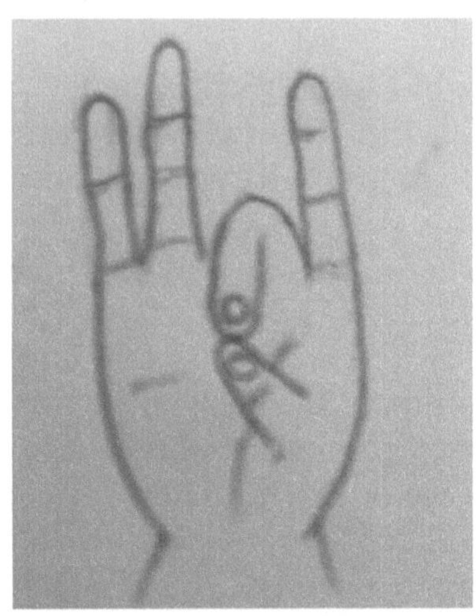

Practice:
1. Posture:
   o   Sit in a comfortable position on chair with your spine straight and shoulders relaxed.
   o   Maintain an upright posture, keeping your head aligned with your spine.

2. Hand Placement:
   o   Fold your middle finger and gently touch it to the tip of your thumb.
   o   Keep the index, ring, and little fingers extended and relaxed.
   o   Rest your hands on your knees or thighs with the palms facing upward or relaxed in your lap.
3. Breathing:
   o   Practice deep, slow breathing, inhaling through the nose and exhaling through the nose.
   o   Focus on your breath to enhance the calming effects of the mudra.
4. Duration:
   o   Hold the mudra for 3-10 minutes, focusing on your breath and the calming sensation it brings.

o   It can be practiced multiple times throughout the day, especially when you feel mentally overwhelmed or stressed.

Benefits of Shuni Mudra for IT Professionals
1. Enhances Concentration and Focus:
o   Shuni Mudra is known to increase mental clarity and focus, which is especially beneficial for IT professionals who need to stay attentive and sharp while coding or working through complex problems.
2. Promotes Patience and Discipline:
o   This mudra cultivates patience, a quality that can help IT professionals stay calm and composed during stressful situations, whether dealing with deadlines, technical challenges, or long work hours.
3. Throat and Saturn Energy get balanced:
o   Shuni Mudra is associated with the throat chakra and the energy of Saturn, which is believed to bring discipline, responsibility, and wisdom.
o   It can help you stay focused on your tasks and encourage clear communication during team collaborations.
4. Reduces Anxiety and Stress:
o   Practicing Shuni Mudra can alleviate mental stress, anxiety, and emotional tension.
o   It helps to calm the nervous system, making it easier to handle high-pressure work environments in tech fields.
5. Improves Patience for Problem-Solving:
o   This mudra helps build emotional resilience and patience, which is particularly useful when faced with long hours of debugging, troubleshooting, or solving complex technical issues.
6. Enhances Emotional Stability:
o   Shuni Mudra promotes emotional stability, preventing feelings of frustration and overwhelm, which are common in fast-paced, challenging work settings.

Chapter 6

Meditation on chair

Meditation

Meditation is a process of training the mind to gain control and focus. It is a science that systematically guides the mind toward greater awareness and clarity. Meditation is a practice that involves focusing attention, calming the mind, and fostering mindfulness. It encourages relaxation, reduces stress, and enhances overall well-being. For IT professionals, regular meditation provides a much-needed mental reset, boosting clarity, creativity, and emotional stability. Meditation bring down the frequency of mind wave.

Why Meditation is Essential for IT Professionals?

Professionals often experience:

- Cognitive Overload: Intense problem-solving, debugging, and coding can lead to mental fatigue.
- Stress and Anxiety: Tight deadlines, constant communication, and multitasking create chronic stress.
- Lack of Focus: Frequent distractions and long working hours can reduce concentration.
- Eye and Neck Strain: Prolonged screen time leads to physical tension and discomfort.
- Sleep Issues: Work-related anxiety can disrupt sleep patterns.

Benefits of Meditation:

- Reduces Stress and Anxiety: Activates the relaxation response, lowering cortisol levels.
- Enhances Focus: Improves attention span and cognitive clarity.

- Promotes Emotional Balance: Helps manage frustration, irritability, and burnout.
- Improves Sleep: Calms the mind, making it easier to fall and stay asleep.
- Boosts Creativity: Encourages divergent thinking and problem-solving skills.
- Reduces Physical Tension: Eases muscle strain and eye fatigue.

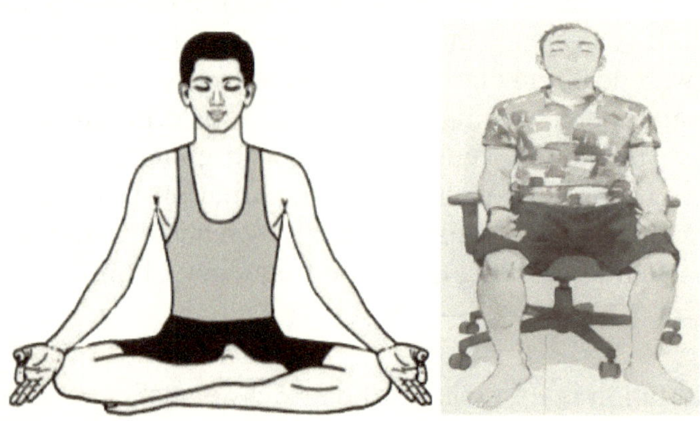

Meditation Techniques for IT Professionals

1. **Mindfulness Meditation**

Goal: To enhance present-moment awareness and reduce mental clutter.

1. Posture:
   - Sit in a chair with your feet flat on the ground and your back straight.
   - Rest your hands on your thighs or in your lap.
   - Close your eyes gently or soften your gaze.

Option:

You can also sit on floor.

2. Breathing:
- o   Take a few deep breaths in through your nose and out through your mouth.
- o   Allow your breathing to settle into a natural rhythm.
3. Awareness:
- o   Focus on the sensation of your breath as it enters and exits your nostrils or the rise and fall of your chest.
- o   If your mind wanders (which is normal), gently return your attention to your breath.
4. Body Scan:
- o   Gradually bring your awareness to different parts of your body, starting from your toes to moving upward to your head.
- o   Notice any tension and consciously release it.
5. Duration:
- o   Practice for 5-10 minutes during a work break or at the end of the day.

2. Focused Attention Meditation

Goal: To sharpen concentration and improve cognitive function.

1. Posture:
- o   Sit comfortably with your back straight and hands resting on your knees.
2. Breathing:
- o   Take a few slow, deep breaths to center yourself.
3. Focus Object:
- o   Choose a simple focal point like:
    - ▪ The sensation of your breath.
    - ▪ A visual object (e.g., a candle flame).
    - ▪ A calming word or phrase (e.g., "Calm" or "Peace").
4. Practice:
- o   Direct all your attention to your chosen focus.
- o   If your mind wanders, gently bring it back without judgment.
5. Duration:
- o   Practice for 5-10 minutes to reset your focus during or after work.

3. Loving-Kindness Meditation (Metta Meditation)

Goal: To cultivate compassion, patience, and emotional balance.

1. Posture:
o   Sit comfortably and close your eyes.
2. Breathing:
o   Take slow, deep breaths to center yourself.
3. Repeat Affirmations:

o   Silently repeat these phrases:
o   For Yourself: "May I be happy. May I be healthy. May I be safe. May I live with ease."
o   For a Colleague: "May my all colleagues be happy. May my all colleagues be healthy. May my all colleagues be safe. May my all colleagues live with ease."
o   For All Beings: "May all beings be happy. May all beings be healthy. May all beings be safe. May all beings live with ease."

4. Duration:
o   Practice for 5-10 minutes to cultivate empathy and reduce workplace tension.

4. Guided Visualization Meditation

Goal: To reduce stress and promote relaxation through mental imagery.

1. Posture:
o   Sit or lie down comfortably.
2. Breathing:
o   Take a few deep breaths to relax your body.
3. Visualization:
o   Imagine a peaceful place (e.g., a forest, beach, or meadow or the early morning round Sun rise).
o   Engage your senses: visualize the sights, sounds, and smells of this place.

o   Feel the relaxation spreading through your body.
4. Duration:
o   Practice for 5-10 minutes to reset your mind during breaks.

Quick 5-Minute Desk Meditation

1. Sit Comfortably:
o   Close your eyes and straighten your back.
2. Deep Breaths:
o   Inhale for 4 counts, hold for 4, exhale for 4 counts.
3. Focus on Breath:
o   Notice the sensation of air flowing in and out.
4. Release Tension:
o   On each exhale, release tension in your body.

Start practicing meditation at least 2 minutes every day and gradually increase the time. Morning time is the best time but can be practice any time when it permits for you in a day.

Closing Prayer

ॐ सर्वेभवन्तुसुखिनः सर्वेसन्तुनिरामयाः ।
सर्वेभद्राणिपश्यन्तुमाकश्चिद्दुःख भाग्भवेत् ।
ॐशान्तिः शान्तिः शान्तिः ॥

Om SarveBhavantuSukhinahSarveSantuNiraamayaah |
SarveBhadraanniPashyantuMaaKashcid-Duhkha-Bhaag-Bhavet |
Om Shaantih Shaantih Shaantih ||

Meaning:
1. Om, May All be Happy,

2. May All be Free from Illness.

3. May All See What Auspicious is,

4. May no one Suffer.

5. Om Peace, Peace, Peace.

References:

1. Iyengar, B. K. S. (2005). Light on Yoga.
2. Bihar School of yoga(Various). magazine, apps, books.
3. S-VYASA Publications (Various). Books on Yoga and Research.
4. Online Resources (Various). Articles, studies, and materials on Yoga.
5. WCSC Vethathiri Publications (Various). Books on Yoga and Spiritual Science.

About the Author:

Jayanta Sarkar, MCA, YIC(Yoga Instructor course), M.Sc. in Yoga For Human Excellence is an experienced IT professional with over 18 years in the tech industry. Balancing long hours at a desk, he discovered the transformative power of yoga and has been practicing for more than 15 years. His deep interest in holistic well-being led him to explore seated yoga techniques that seamlessly integrate into a busy professional's routine.

Passionate about making yoga accessible to working individuals, Jayanta combines his expertise in mindfulness, breathwork, and posture correction to help others cultivate clarity, calmness, and vitality-right at their desks. He is currently pursuing a Ph.D. in Yoga and continues to research innovative ways to bridge ancient yogic wisdom with modern work-life challenges.

When he's not coding or teaching yoga, Jayanta enjoys exploring spiritual texts, writing about wellness, and sharing his knowledge to empower professionals worldwide.